TABLE OF CONTENTS

Top 20 Test Taking Tips

1. Carefully follow all the test registration procedures
2. Know the test directions, duration, topics, question types, how many questions
3. Setup a flexible study schedule at least 3-4 weeks before test day
4. Study during the time of day you are most alert, relaxed, and stress free
5. Maximize your learning style; visual learner use visual study aids, auditory learner use auditory study aids
6. Focus on your weakest knowledge base
7. Find a study partner to review with and help clarify questions
8. Practice, practice, practice
9. Get a good night's sleep; don't try to cram the night before the test
10. Eat a well balanced meal
11. Know the exact physical location of the testing site; drive the route to the site prior to test day
12. Bring a set of ear plugs; the testing center could be noisy
13. Wear comfortable, loose fitting, layered clothing to the testing center; prepare for it to be either cold or hot during the test
14. Bring at least 2 current forms of ID to the testing center
15. Arrive to the test early; be prepared to wait and be patient
16. Eliminate the obviously wrong answer choices, then guess the first remaining choice
17. Pace yourself; don't rush, but keep working and move on if you get stuck
18. Maintain a positive attitude even if the test is going poorly
19. Keep your first answer unless you are positive it is wrong
20. Check your work, don't make a careless mistake

Be Aware

1. You only have to get about 55-65% of the questions right to pass in many cases depending on the difficulty of the test.
2. 300 questions offered on the PANCE test.
3. Each area of basic knowledge is not included with a specific block. All of the material is random. You will be required to "switch gears" between each of the above content areas.
4. The PANCE is offered on the computer.
5. Make sure you are registered for the exam. Go to: http://www.nccpa.net to register.

PANCE Score Reporting

Generally, test scores are repored back to the student within a 2 week time period. All scores are compared to a test group selected by test writers. A passing score on the test is around 55%-65% correct answers on most exams. The key testing score is a pass/fail analysis. Basically, you either pass or fail.

Organ System

Cardiovascular

Dilated cardiomyopathy

Dilated cardiomyopathy is the most common type of cardiomyopathy. It results in a reduction in strength of the ventricular contraction, which causes dilation of the left ventricle and a decreased ejection fraction. Most common causes are alcohol abuse, cocaine abuse, CAD, thyroid disease, and pheochromocytoma, but it can also be due to an autoimmune or infective process. Infective myocarditis due to the coxsackievirus can lead to dilated cardiomyopathy.

Symptoms and diagnosis

Dilated cardiomyopathy will cause patients to feel short of breath, and paroxysmal nocturnal dyspnea may be present with complaints of fatigue. As the ejection fraction decreases, symptoms of CHF may be present, such as rales, edema, a systolic murmur, and an increase in jugular venous distention (JVD). The murmur heard with dilated cardiomyopathy should decrease when patients are standing or performing Valsalva maneuvers.

An EKG will show ST-T wave changes with left ventricular hypertrophy and possible conduction abnormalities. A chest x-ray will show cardiomegaly and possible pulmonary congestion and effusions. An echocardiogram will assess valvular function and estimate the ejection fraction. If there is an autoimmune or infective process present, a myocardial biopsy will be done to identify the causative factor. A cardiac catheterization can be done to determine the extent of CAD present, and lab work will be done to identify if there is an endocrine abnormality. Finally, a urine or serum drug screen will identify if illicit drug use is the cause of the heart disease.

Restrictive cardiomyopathy

Restrictive cardiomyopathy occurs due to some type of infiltrative process that results in decreased elasticity of the ventricles and heart failure. It can be idiopathic in nature or due to conditions that result in endomyocardial fibrosis, such as sarcoidosis or amyloidosis.

Symptoms and diagnosis

Restrictive cardiomyopathy may also cause dyspnea and fatigue with paroxysmal nocturnal dyspnea. Edema, rales, and an increase in jugular venous distention may also be present. A heart murmur may be auscultated, and patients may have chronic atrial fibrillation. The murmur heard with restrictive cardiomyopathy should decrease when patients are standing or performing Valsalva maneuvers.

An echocardiogram will be done to confirm the diagnosis of restrictive cardiomyopathy. This will show restriction of the heart movements with a decrease in the estimated ejection fraction. Though this can be idiopathic in etiology, a myocardial biopsy will be done to determine the cause. It would be expected that evidence of sarcoidosis or amyloidosis would be present on biopsy if either of these is the cause. Collagen deposits may also be present when collagen disease is the cause of the restrictive cardiomyopathy. Many tests will be done to confirm a diagnosis of these disorders if they are thought to be the cause.

Hypertrophic cardiomyopathy

Hypertrophic cardiomyopathy causes a significant enlargement of the left ventricle, especially the septum, which results in obstruction of the left ventricle. This is most often genetic in etiology and can be seen in young athletes. Hypertension may also contribute to development of this type of cardiomyopathy.

Symptoms and diagnosis

Hypertrophic cardiomyopathy may not give any warning signs to patients and is frequently the cause of sudden cardiac arrest in the young athlete. If symptomatic, patients may complain of dyspnea on exertion, angina, palpitations, fatigue, or episodes of syncope. A systolic murmur can be heard with hypertrophic cardiomyopathy, but unlike the other types of cardiomyopathy, the intensity of the murmur will not change when patients are standing or performing Valsalva maneuvers.

EKG changes seen with hypertrophic cardiomyopathy include ST-T wave changes, left ventricular hypertrophy, and deep Q waves. An echocardiogram will be done to assess valvular function and the estimated ejection fraction. Patients may undergo cardiac catheterization to assess for CAD. A Holter monitor may be worn by patients to assess for any variations in heart rate or rhythm during a specific time period. Because hypertrophic cardiomyopathy tends to be a genetic condition, patients' families should undergo a thorough cardiac evaluation.

EKG results

Atrial fibrillation and treatment

Atrial fibrillation on EKG results in an irregularly irregular rhythm with no visible P waves. The QRX complex is usually ≤ 0.12 seconds. With atrial fibrillation, there are multiple sites within the atria that are initiating electrical impulses for cardiac contraction. Because of this, the atria are not contracting on a regular basis, resulting in an irregular ventricular response.

If patients are stable and this is new onset atrial fibrillation (<48 hours), diltiazem or beta-blockers can be used to decrease the heart rate. Chemical cardioversion can be performed by administering amiodarone or digoxin, or electrical cardioversion can be performed with patients sedated.

If patients are stable, but it is not known how long they have been in atrial fibrillation, full anticoagulation should be performed and a transesophageal echocardiogram should be done to assess for atrial thrombus before any chemical or electrical cardioversion is performed. If the heart rate is >150 and patients are unstable, immediate synchronized cardioversion should be done to normalize the rate.

Atrial flutter and treatment

Atrial flutter on EKG results in a regular rhythm with an atrial rate up to 300 bpm. The P waves will follow a "sawtooth" pattern two or more times followed by a narrow QRS. A bundle branch block may be present, and this can result in a widened QRS. This occurs when the atrial focus is irritated, resulting in multiple firings. The AV node will block some of these impulses from being sent to the ventricles. This can cause the ventricular rhythm to be normal or abnormal.

If patients with atrial flutter are stable, diltiazem or a beta-blocker can be used to decrease the heart rate. Chemical cardioversion with amiodarone or digoxin can be used to normalize the rate, or electrical cardioversion can be performed while patients are sedated. If the heart rate is >150 and patients are unstable, immediate synchronized cardioversion should be performed.

1st-degree AV block

- 1st-degree AV block occurs when there is a delay in the transmission of the electrical impulse in the heart from the SA node to the AV node. This does not result in a change in the heart rate, but the EKG will exhibit a lengthened PR interval to >0.2 seconds. There should be regular P waves followed by a QRS complex and the rhythm should be regular. The rest of the EKG should be normal, and patients should be in normal sinus rhythm.
- 1st-degree AV block does not cause symptoms in patients, and no treatment is necessary. If patients have an underlying condition that could be contributing to the 1st-degree AV block, such as hypoxia, MI, or dehydration, then those conditions should be treated appropriately. The most likely cause for 1st-degree AV block is an electrical problem in the AV node itself, and it is more likely to develop in the elderly.

2nd-degree AV block

Second-degree AV block can be categorized as type 1 or type 2.

- Type 1 2nd-degree AV block occurs when the time it takes for the electrical impulse to travel from the SA node to the AV node increases in length until a ventricular beat is finally skipped. On the EKG, this will look like a gradually increasing PR interval until a QRS is dropped. This can be treated with atropine if it results in symptomatic bradycardia or pacing can normalize the rate.
- Type 2 2nd degree AV block occurs when the electrical impulse signal travels from the SA node to the AV node, but the signal does not always continue onto the ventricles to cause a contraction. On EKG, this results in a normal PR interval and QRS or a normal PR interval and absent QRS. This is treated with pacing, and transcutaneous pacing may be necessary if patients are clinically unstable.

3rd-degree AV block

Third degree AV block is considered complete heart block. The SA node continues to send its electrical impulse to the AV node, but the AV node is not transmitting this signal onto the ventricles. The ventricles are contracting, but this contraction is due to stimulation of the ventricular fibers so the heart rate is usually decreased to <40 bpm. On EKG, this results in regularly-occurring P waves and regularly-occurring QRS complexes that are completely independently of each other. The atrial rate is normal at 60-100 bpm, but the ventricular rate will be bradycardic. The QRS complexes may appear wide.

Myocardial infarction resulting in cardiac hypoxia can cause a disruption in the electrical system of the heart by damaging the AV node so the impulse cannot be transmitted from the SA node to the ventricles.

This condition requires transcutaneous pacing until permanent pacing can be established. Dopamine and IV fluids may also be given. Patients should be monitored for a change in symptoms.

Premature atrial contractions

With a premature atrial contraction (PAC), there is an area within the atria that is irritated and is triggering delivery of sporadic impulses. This results in the atria contracting at a time out of sync with the regular rhythm of the atria. On EKG, P waves may be present, but extra P waves may be hidden within the QRS complex or T waves. The QRS is usually narrow unless a bundle branch block that causes it to be widened is present.

Premature atrial contractions are generally not symptomatic and not considered dangerous. Many people have these occurring and do not know it, but some patients may feel a palpitation in their chest when premature atrial contractions occur. They do not require any treatment unless there is an underlying problem that needs to be treated. Usually the cause is unknown, but these could occur due to an irritation in the heart's electrical system.

Bundle branch block

A bundle branch block (BBB) can occur within the left or right ventricle. It is usually due to an area of muscle damage. As the electrical impulse travels from the atria to the ventricles, the undamaged ventricle will transmit the signal normally. The damaged ventricle, however, will be delayed in transmitting the signal and this will result in two QRS complexes on EKG.

A quick way to diagnose a patient with a bundle branch block is to look at the V1, V2, V5, and V6 leads. With a right BBB, the V1 and V2 leads will exhibit an abnormal QRS complex with a "rabbit ears" appearance. With a left BBB, leads V5 and V6 will exhibit a widened QRS complex with a notched appearance.

A left or right bundle branch block does not require treatment. It is important to remember, however, that a patient with clinical symptoms representing an acute MI cannot be diagnosed with an MI by EKG alone if a bundle branch block is present.

Paroxysmal supraventricular tachycardia

Paroxysmal supraventricular tachycardia (PVST) is an elevated heart rate that originates within the atria. The rate is so fast that the underlying rhythm cannot be diagnosed. The heart rate is usually >150 bpm and regular. On EKG, P waves are usually not present, or they are buried behind the QRS complex. The PR interval cannot be determined because of the absence of P wave, and QRS complex is usually very narrow.

If patients have a heart rate >150 but are clinically stable, vagal maneuvers can sometimes help to convert the rate to sinus rhythm. Adenosine 6 mg IV can also be given. If this does not work, this can be followed by adenosine 12 mg IV and a second dose of 12 mg if necessary. If the underlying rhythm can be determined, that can be treated appropriately.

If patients have a rate of >150 bpm and is unstable, immediate electrical synchronized cardioversion is necessary to attempt to return to sinus rhythm.

Premature ventricular contractions

Premature ventricular contractions (PVCs) occur when there is an area of irritability within a ventricle, causing it to contract early. This will result in a "missed beat" in the heart rate. The heart rate can vary and will depend upon the underlying rhythm. PVCs generally cause an irregular heart rate, but there can be regularity present if bigeminy is present. This occurs when PVC is present after every regular ventricular beat. Trigeminy occurs when PVC occurs during every third ventricular beat.

On EKG, the QRS will appear abnormal with a much-widened QRS complex. The pattern of bigeminy or trigeminy may be present. P waves are not present before the widened QRS.

Treatment of PVCs involves treating the underlying cause. Oxygen can help to decrease the PVCs, but antiarrhythmic medications (Lidocaine, etc.) may be necessary if the PVCs are frequent to reduce the risk of ventricular tachycardia or ventricular fibrillation.

Ventricular tachycardia

Ventricular tachycardia occurs when the ventricles repeatedly contract without the atria contracting. This can be a deadly arrhythmia and is considered a cardiac emergency. On EKG, all that will be seen are tall, widened QRS complexes. The rate is usually regular at around 150 up to 250 bpm. No P waves are present.

Though patients may appear stable and conscious, this will not last long. Antiarrhythmics, such as amiodarone and lidocaine, should be given to convert to sinus rhythm. Patients should be given IV fluids, also, and dopamine may be given at 5-20 μg/kg/min. ACLS protocol should be followed, including unsynchronized cardioversion/defibrillation to attempt to convert to sinus rhythm.

A magnesium deficiency can cause a form of ventricular tachycardia called *torsades de pointes.* This will appear as a series of widened QRS complexes that vary in height in a wave pattern. Magnesium should be given to attempt to convert to sinus rhythm.

Ventricular fibrillation

Ventricular fibrillation occurs when the ventricles are in a state of uncontrolled spasm, like quivering, without being able to complete a forceful contraction. This is considered a true cardiac arrest with no organized electrical activity.

On EKG, the heart rate will not be able to be determined because of the irregularity. No P waves will be discernible, and no organized QRS complexes will be present. The rhythm can appear to be coarse or fine. Ventricular fibrillation can resemble artifact so the leads must be placed correctly on patients, especially if patients are alert and stable while this rhythm appears to be present.

ACLS protocol should be followed for treatment of ventricular fibrillation. Immediate unsynchronized cardioversion/defibrillation should be provided. Antiarrhythmics, such as amiodarone, lidocaine, or magnesium should be given. Dopamine may also be given at a rate of 5-20 μg/kg/min. Patients should be well oxygenated or intubated to ensure oxygen needs are being met.

Ventricular flutter

Ventricular flutter is very similar to ventricular fibrillation; however, there is even less unorganized ventricular activity. The ventricles will spasm without any discernible pattern of organized activity. This arrhythmia is usually short-lived and is not present for a long period of time.

On EKG, the heart rate will not be able to be determined because of the irregularity. No P waves will be discernible and no organized QRS complexes will be present. The rhythm can appear to be coarse or fine. Ventricular flutter can resemble artifact, so the leads must be placed correctly on patients, especially if patients are alert and stable while this rhythm appears to be present.

ACLS protocol should be followed for treatment of ventricular flutter. Immediate unsynchronized cardioversion/defibrillation should be provided. Antiarrhythmics, such as amiodarone, lidocaine, or magnesium should be given. Dopamine may also be given at a rate of 5-20 μg/kg/min. Patients should be well oxygenated or intubated to ensure oxygen needs are being met.

Atrial septal defect

An atrial septal defect is a congenital heart defect in which there is an opening between the left and right atrium. This results in failure to thrive in the infant. The infant will exhibit dyspnea, clubbing of the nails, and excessive fatigue. On exam, a systolic murmur and a widely split and fixed S_2 will be heard. EKG findings will include atrial fibrillation, with a right bundle branch block and a right axis deviation.

An atrial septal defect is diagnosed initially through a combination of exam findings and EKG changes. An echocardiogram and an angiogram will be done to confirm the diagnosis. This is not diagnosed *in utero* because of the presence of the patent foramen ovale. It is usually detected within a couple of days of birth.

Treatment is now being done using cardiac catheterization techniques to patch the defect, though open surgery is the most commonly-used form of treatment.

Coarctation of the aorta

Coarctation of the aorta is a congenital heart defect in which there is narrowing of the aorta distal to the left subclavian artery. This results in the development of collateral circulation through the intercostal arteries and the branches of the subclavian artery. It is most common in male children and is often associated with Turner's syndrome in females.

Clinically, the infant may exhibit hypertension with varying blood pressure between the upper and lower extremities. The pulses may also vary between the two sets of extremities. Symptoms of congestive heart failure may be present along with weak or absent femoral pulses. A systolic murmur will be heard predominantly over the back.

Coarctation of the aorta is diagnosed using a chest x-ray in which rib notching will be evident due to the development of collateral vessels trying to pass over the coarctation. An EKG and echocardiogram will also be done. Diagnosis is confirmed using angiogram.

Treatments include balloon angioplasty to attempt to widen the aorta. Open surgery may need to be performed.

Patent ductus arteriosus

Patent ductus arteriosus is a congenital heart defect in which the ductus arteriosus fails to close after birth. The ductus arteriosus is an opening, present *in utero*, that serves as a shunt between the left pulmonary artery and the aorta. This opening can fail to close due to a rubella infection while *in utero.*

Clinically, the infant will exhibit pulmonary hypertension and a failure to thrive. On exam, there will be a continuous machinery murmur heard. A thrill may be palpated over the chest wall and the back. A widened pulse pressure will also be present.

Patent ductus arteriosus is diagnosed through a combination of exam findings, EKG, echocardiogram, and chest x-ray, but is confirmed by angiogram. It is diagnosed within a couple of days of birth. Closure of the ductus arteriosus can usually be achieved using less invasive cardiac catheterization techniques, but open surgery may be necessary.

Tetralogy of Fallot

Tetralogy of Fallot is a congenital heart defect that comprises four conditions: a ventricular septal defect, overriding of the aorta, right ventricular hypertrophy, and right ventricular outflow obstruction (pulmonary stenosis). This is the most common cyanotic infant heart disease and the least understood. There are likely genetic factors associated with the development of this condition. There may also be some medications taken by the mother during pregnancy that can result in Tetralogy of Fallot in the fetus.

Clinically, the infant will be cyanotic with dyspnea and clubbing. A holosystolic murmur can be heard on exam. This condition can result in retarded growth in childhood. Tetralogy of Fallot can be diagnosed using EKG, echocardiogram, and angiogram. A CBC will show polycythemia.

Surgery is necessary to treat Tetralogy of Fallot. Patients will always require endocarditis prophylaxis before all dental procedures and other invasive procedures throughout their lifetimes.

Ventricular septal defect

A ventricular septal defect is a congenital heart defect in which there is an opening between the left and right ventricles. There is no known cause of this condition, but it probably occurs during development of the heart *in utero*. This condition can be associated with Eisenmenger's syndrome.

Clinically, the infant will exhibit signs of pulmonary hypertension and congestive heart failure. Very rapid respirations may be present with sweating and pallor. The infant may have great difficulty eating because of the difficulty breathing, resulting in the failure to gain weight and failure to thrive. On exam, a holosystolic murmur can be heard, and a systolic thrill may be palpated over the chest wall and back.

A ventricular septal defect is diagnosed using exam findings, echocardiogram, chest x-ray, and angiogram. An EKG will show a right bundle branch block.

Closure of the ventricular septal defect can be attempted using cardiac catheterization techniques, but open surgery may be necessary.

Essential, secondary, and malignant hypertension

- Essential hypertension is the most common form of hypertension. The cause of this type of hypertension is unknown. Most patients are also unaware that they are suffering from hypertension with this type. It is diagnosed after patients have three separate episodes of blood pressure 140/90 or higher, not found to be due to some type of medical condition.
- Secondary hypertension only affects about 5% of the population of patients who have been diagnosed with hypertension. It is due to another medical condition, such as renal disease (most common), renal artery stenosis, aldosteronism, or pheochromocytoma.
- Malignant hypertension is uncontrolled severe hypertension and can be life-threatening. It can be due to secondary causes (renal artery stenosis) or the cause may be unknown. The goal with malignant hypertension is to provide immediate treatment by decreasing the blood pressure slowly, no more than 25% over 1-2 hours. Nitroprusside, nitroglycerin, labetalol, and clonidine are the most common medications used to treat this condition.

Hypertension in adults

The standard classifications of hypertension in adults are as follows:

Classification	Systolic BP mm Hg	Diastolic BP mm Hgb
Normal	< 120	And < 80
Pre-hypertension	120 – 139	Or 80 – 89
Stage 1 hypertension	140-159	Or 90 – 99
Stage 2 hypertension	≥ 160	Or ≥ 100

Managing hypertension

Beta-blockers

Beta-blockers help to lower blood pressure by decreasing the heart rate and the force that is exerted by the ventricles with each heartbeat. Beta-blockers work on beta-receptors, though not all beta-blockers are created to work just on cardiac beta-receptors. Some of these medications, especially the older medications, work on all the beta-receptors in the body. Beta-blockers are now thought to help extend life in patients with known CAD, those who have had an MI, and those patients with known CHF.

Because beta-blockers reduce the heart rate, there is a risk that they can cause the heart rate and blood pressure to drop too low. This can result in dizziness, confusion, and possibly even syncope. There is a small risk of erectile dysfunction when beta-blockers are used by male patients.

Some examples of beta-blockers include metoprolol (Lopressor®), atenolol (Tenormin®), and carvedilol (Coreg®).

Diuretics

Diuretics work on the kidneys to increase the amount of water and sodium that are excreted from the body through the urine. This helps to reduce the actual fluid volume in the body, thus decreasing the amount of pressure within the arteries and resulting in a lowered blood pressure. Because diuretics work on the kidneys, they may not be appropriate for all patients, especially those with renal disease.

Along with the water and sodium that is increasingly excreted from the body, potassium is also depleted with some of the diuretics. This can result in hypokalemia in some patients, so a potassium supplement is often prescribed along with the diuretic. Eating foods high in potassium may also help patients prevent a decrease in potassium levels. An increase in urinary frequency is frequently seen, so patients should take diuretics in the morning to prevent having to get up frequently during the night.

Examples of some diuretics include furosemide (Lasix®), hydrochlorothiazide, spironolactone (Aldactone®), and torsemide (Demadex®).

ACE inhibitors

ACE inhibitors work on the arteries to cause dilation, which decreases the pressure within the arteries and leads to a decrease in blood pressure. Their effects also help patients with congestive heart failure by potentially preventing hospitalizations, decreasing the risk of a future MI, and decreasing the risk of death due to CHF.

Because ACE inhibitors cause arterial dilation, they can, in rare cases, cause angioedema. This results when there is an excessive dilation in the arteries of the lips and face. Though rare, this type of allergic reaction is a medical emergency and should be treated immediately. The most common potential side effect of ACE inhibitors is a chronic, nonproductive cough. This can be very annoying to patients and may be a reason for noncompliance in those who develop the cough. ACE inhibitors may cause the kidneys to decrease excretion of potassium, so patients should be monitored for hyperkalemia.

Some examples of ACE inhibitors include captopril (Capoten®), enalapril (Vasotec®), and quinapril (Accupril®).

Angiotensin-receptor blockers
Angiotensin-receptor blockers (ARBs) work the same as ACE inhibitors as they work on the arteries to cause dilation, which decreases the pressure within the arteries and leads to a decrease in blood pressure. Their effects also help patients with congestive heart failure by potentially preventing hospitalizations, decreasing the risk of a future MI, and decreasing the risk of death due to CHF.

The reason that an ARB may be prescribed instead of an ACE inhibitor is because of a lesser risk of side effects. Patients who suffer from side effects with ACE inhibitors, especially the chronic cough, may tolerate ARBs without any difficulties. Though side effects are rare with ARBs, kidney function should be monitored.

Examples of ARBs include losartan (Cozaar®), telmisartan (Micardis®), and valsartan (Diovan®).

Calcium channel blockers
The older calcium channel blockers work in two different ways. They dilate the arteries, thus decreasing the pressure within the arteries, resulting in a decrease in blood pressure. They also decrease the heart rate and decrease the force of ventricular contractions. The new calcium channel blockers only work to cause arterial dilation.

Patients who suffer from pulmonary hypertension should not be given calcium channel blockers if it can be avoided. These medications may worsen that condition and could have life-threatening affects. The older calcium channel blockers that cause a decrease in ventricular force may worsen CHF in those patients who suffer from this illness. Most of the calcium channel blockers can potentially cause headaches and peripheral edema.

Examples of older calcium channel blockers include diltiazem (Cardizem®) and verapamil (Calan®). New calcium channel blockers include amlodipine (Norvasc®) and felodipine (Plendil®).

Cardiogenic shock

Cardiogenic shock is a condition in which the heart is not able to supply the body with the necessary blood, oxygen, and nutrients that are necessary for proper functioning and survival. It can be caused by damage to the heart muscle itself, resulting in decreased effectiveness of pumping, disruption in the electrical system of the heart that result in inadequate cardiac contractility, or valvular abnormalities that prevent the proper flow of blood through the heart.

If alert, patients may complain of a feeling of anxiety and breathlessness, heart palpitations, or weakness and fatigue. Patients may appear visibly pale or mottled in color with restlessness or lethargy leading to coma. Urine output may be decreased, or patients may not have any measurable urine output.

This condition is fatal approximately 80% of the time. Treatment is immediate with medications to help raise the blood pressure and improve cardiac function. This includes epinephrine, dobutamine, dopamine, and norepinephrine. Cardiac pacing may be necessary.

Orthostatic hypotension

Orthostatic hypotension is a sudden drop in blood pressure that is symptomatic. It usually occurs when a patient stands up quickly or is rising from a lying to sitting or standing position. Medications are the most common cause of orthostatic hypotension, including antihypertensives, antianxiety drugs, and diuretics. Excessive alcohol use can also cause orthostatic hypotension.

Patients will describe a sudden dizziness or light-headed sensation when moving too quickly, usually rising from sitting or lying down. This can be severe enough to cause syncope or near-syncopal episodes. Some patients may describe nausea with this sensation.

Patients should be advised to avoid any rapid movements. They should rise slowly from a sitting or lying position. Sitting at the edge of the bed for a few minutes before standing up can prevent the sudden drop in blood pressure upon standing. If orthostatic hypotension is persistent, the cause should be treated. This may involve trying other medications to treat an underlying medical condition if medications are the cause of this condition.

Acute myocardial infarction

Patients may complain of a crushing pressure throughout the chest, radiating into the neck or left arm. They may also have epigastric pain or a feeling of weakness or anxiety. Elderly patients and diabetics may not have any of the classic symptoms of an acute MI.

Objectively, patients may be pale and diaphoretic. They may appear restless or lethargic. On exam, an S_4 gallop may be heard. Blood pressure may be high or low. Acute symptoms of CHF may be seen.

EKG may show ST elevation, though depression can also be seen. Cardiac enzymes should be drawn every 8 hours x 3. Troponin 1 is usually the first enzyme that is elevated, followed by CKMB. Evaluate the CKMB percentage to ensure there is an elevation. A 5-10% elevation in the CKMB most likely indicates ischemia. Higher elevations are indicative of an acute MI. An echocardiogram may show a decreased ejection fraction. Cardiac wall stiffness may be seen if there is an S_4 gallop.

Treatments

Remember the pneumonic: nurse MONA has great ABs. This stands for MI treatment with morphine, oxygen, nitrates, aspirin, ACE inhibitors, and beta-blockers. If the diagnosis of an acute MI is confirmed, thrombolytic ("clot buster") medications may be given to open the blocked coronary artery. These can have serious side effects and a careful assessment of patients' medical history should be done before considering these medications.

Ideally, patients should be stabilized and taken for a cardiac catheterization within 90 minutes of presenting to the ER. Angioplasty can be performed during catheterization, if possible, to open the blocked coronary artery and restore blood flow to the heart muscle. The quicker that blood flow is restored to the heart muscle, the less the risk of permanent muscle damage. A stent may need to be placed to prevent collapse and spasm of the coronary artery. If there is excessive coronary artery disease, coronary artery bypass grafting may need to be considered once patients are stabilized.

Angina pectoris

Angina is chest pain that is usually brought on by stress or exertion and relieved by rest and/or nitrate medications. It can be classified as stable, unstable, or Prinzmetal (variant) type.

- Stable angina lasts < 30 minutes. It is increased with activity and decreased with rest and/or nitrates. It is described as a clenching sensation over the chest and may be accompanied by pallor, diaphoresis, and hypertension.

- Unstable angina can last >30 minutes at rest and symptoms tend to continue after nitrates are taken. Patients will notice that the episodes are becoming more frequent and lasting longer. It may be associated with symptoms of CHF, and new EKG changes of increasing ST depression may be seen.
- Prinzmetal's (variant) angina is due to a spasm of the coronary arteries. It occurs more often in men than women. It usually occurs during rest without any specific triggering activity. It is usually relieved by nitrates. Though rare, an acute MI could occur during an episode of coronary artery spasm.

Acute rheumatic fever

Acute rheumatic fever can occur approximately 2 weeks following a pharynx infection with β-hemolytic *Streptococcus*. It usually affects children 5 to 15 years old and is no longer common in the United States. Approximately 75% of cases will affect the mitral valve and 30% affect the aortic valve.

In order to diagnose rheumatic fever, at least 2 of the Jones criteria must be present: carditis, erythema marginatum, subcutaneous nodules, Sydenham's chorea, or migratory arthritis of the large joints.

Along with the Jones criteria, patients will have a fever. They may complain of polyarthralgia. An EKG will show a prolonged PR interval. Abnormal lab tests will include an elevation in erythrocyte sedimentation rate (ESR) and throat cultures positive for Strep.

Rheumatic fever can be deadly and lead to permanent heart disease, CHF, arrhythmias, and pericardial effusions. Treatment includes bed rest, penicillin, and steroids. Haldol may be given to control the movements of chorea.

Aortic aneurysm

An aortic aneurysm is a dilation of the aorta >3 cm. It is usually seen at a level below the renal arteries but can be common in the thoracic aorta in patients who have Marfan's syndrome. Those who are most at risk for developing an aortic aneurysm are men >60-years-old who smoke and have hypertension. Most patients with an aortic aneurysm are asymptomatic unless dissection or rupture occurs. Patients may have complaints of vague back pain before dissection or rupture occurs.

Clinically, a pulsatile mass may be felt in very thin patients, but an abdominal bruit will be heard over the area before a mass is palpated. If dissection or rupture is suspected, there will be decreased pulses felt below the level of the aneurysm.

Ultrasound or CT/MRI will visualize the aneurysm. Angiography will confirm diagnosis. If a patient has a known aneurysm, an annual ultrasound should be done to monitor its growth. Surgery is usually recommended once it is 5 cm or larger.

Treatment

Patients may know that they have an aortic aneurysm that has been monitored over a period of time. Most aneurysms are asymptomatic, though, so the healthcare provider may not have this information. Patients will describe a fairly sudden onset of mid-abdominal pain that is ripping or tearing in quality. This pain may be aggravated by taking a deep breath or by performing any activities. They may also have severe back pain. Hip pain may also be present if blood is pooling in the lower abdominal cavity.

Clinically, a pulsatile mass may or may not be palpated. It is advised that no hard palpation be performed on the abdomen until an aneurysm is ruled out because of fear of causing sudden rupture if the dissection is advanced. Immediate CT should be done to confirm the diagnosis. Emergency surgery should also be performed because of the very high incidence of death from aortic aneurysm rupture.

Artery and vein disorders

Arterial thrombosis and embolism

An arterial thrombosis is a blood clot located within an artery. This is a stationary clot that can grow large enough to cause occlusion of the vessel. An arterial embolism is the term used for the thrombus once it breaks free and begins moving through the vascular system. This embolism will eventually travel to an artery that is too small to accommodate its size. This results in occlusion of the artery with possible life-threatening results.

Treatment of an arterial thrombus is centered on prevention. Daily aspirin therapy (81 mg) can provide antiplatelet activity that prevents platelets from forming a clot. Other anticoagulant medications, such as Coumadin® and Plavix®, can be used to prevent platelet accumulation and help prevent clot formation. If an arterial thrombus does form and becomes an embolism, treatment is more of an emergency. For example, an arterial embolism is usually a fatal condition, but "clot buster" thrombolytic medications or even surgery to remove the clot may help improve patients' prognosis.

Peripheral arterial disease

Peripheral arterial disease occurs when there is obstruction or narrowing of an artery that interferes with blood flow. This can be due to atherosclerosis, trauma, or inflammation. Patients will frequently complain of pain in their legs or calves after walking a short distance. This pain is relieved with rest. Some male patients may complain about erectile dysfunction. Patients may also state they have numbing and tingling sensations in their extremities.

Clinically, there may be obvious signs of obstructed blood flow, such as pallor, atrophic skin, and hair loss. The peripheral pulses may be decreased or absent if occlusion is present. In severe cases, arterial ulcers may be present with development of gangrene.

Doppler ultrasound will identify decreased blood flow through the arteries. Angiography confirms the diagnosis by providing visualization of the narrowed vessels. Patients should also be assessed for CAD because generally all of the arteries in the body can be affected by this.

Giant cell arteritis

Giant cell arteritis, or temporal arteritis, is an inflammatory process that affects the vessels, most commonly the temporal artery. This condition can lead to occlusion of the temporal artery, resulting in blindness, so diagnosis and treatment should be started quickly.

The most common symptom with giant cell arteritis is a severe headache. This can be accompanied with a fever, generalized body aches, fatigue, or weight loss. Approximately 50% of patients who are diagnosed with giant cell arteritis will also have a diagnosis of polymyalgia rheumatica.

This condition is confirmed by doing a biopsy of the affected vessel, usually the temporal artery. Because of the nature of the illness, treatment is started before the biopsy results are available. Treatment consists of prednisone, usually 40-60 mg per day. This should be continued for at least 1 month and then tapered. If symptoms return as the dose of prednisone is tapered, the dosage can be increased.

Phlebitis

Phlebitis is inflammation that is present in a vein. It is gradual in onset and develops into a reddened, often streaky area that follows the path of a vein. The area may be swollen, indurated, and warm. Patients will often complain of pain in the area. If the phlebitis is superficial, warm compresses, elevation of the affected limb, and compression can help to resolve the problem. If recurrent phlebitis is occurring in the deeper vessels, an anticoagulant may be prescribed to prevent formation of a blood clot.

Thrombophlebitis

Thrombophlebitis occurs when a blood clot forms within the vein, causing inflammation. Patients complain of pain that may be gradual or sudden in onset. It is seen most often in more sedentary patients. The affected area may be red, swollen, or indurated. Patients may have a positive Homan's sign. Treatment consists of anticoagulants to prevent recurrence and to decrease the risk of embolism. Prevention is crucial in treatment with compression stockings, leg elevation, and decreasing the amount of time spent immobile.

Varicose veins

Varicose veins occur due to faulty valves within the distal veins, leading to distention and stretching of the veins. Because the valves are not functioning properly, blood tends to pool in the extremities and cause further distention of the veins.

Patients will complain of aching pain in the legs after standing or sitting for extended periods of time. They may also experience an itching sensation around the veins. If severe, venous stasis ulcers can develop in the lower extremities. The veins will be visibly distended, bulging, and contorted. The skin may appear darkly pigmented due to venous stasis.

The best treatment of varicose veins is prevention. This includes avoiding standing for prolonged periods of time, exercising regularly to keep weight under control, and wearing compression stockings or maintaining leg elevation to promote venous return from the lower extremities. Medical treatments include sclerotherapy, laser vein ablation, vein stripping, or, in severe case, complete removal of the varicose veins.

Aortic stenosis

Aortic stenosis is very common and is the worst valve disease. Most patients are asymptomatic until they reach middle age. Aortic calcifications are frequently seen in those >55-years-old. Aortic stenosis can also be due to a congenital disorder of the bicuspid valve or rheumatic fever.

Patients may have syncopal episodes when aortic stenosis becomes symptomatic. They may complain of chest pain, fatigue, and shortness of breath with activity. Symptoms of CHF can be present when the disease is advanced and prognosis is usually poor by the time these symptoms are present.

On exam, a systolic murmur that is crescendo/decrescendo in nature during the middle to late portion of the cardiac cycle can be heard. This murmur will radiate superiorly to the carotid arteries. There may also be an early systolic ejection click. *Pulsus parvus,* or a weakened pulse, may be palpated. Also, *pulsus tardus,* or a slow-rising pulse may be present.

Aortic insufficiency

Aortic insufficiency can have many causes, including hypertension, rheumatic heart disease, endocarditis, syphilis, and Marfan's syndrome. It can also be congenital in nature.

Patients will complain of fatigue and shortness of breath with activity. The symptoms may be chronic or acute. On exam, a diastolic murmur will be heard, increasing when patients are sitting or holding their breath. A widened pulse pressure will also be detected. Corrigan's sign, a water hammer pulse, may be present. Quincke's pulse, an alternating erythema and paleness in the nail beds with each heartbeat, may also be seen. Musset's sign, patients visibly nodding the head with each heartbeat, may be evident. An Austin flint murmur may be present in severe cases. This murmur sounds like a mid-diastolic, low-pitched rumbling over the cardiac apex. Patients may have all or only a few of these findings.

Mitral stenosis

Mitral stenosis is fairly common, and symptoms will be much more pronounced in females during pregnancy. In rare cases, mitral stenosis is due to rheumatic fever. Patients may complain of hoarseness that will not go away because of recurrent pressure being applied to the laryngeal nerve. Patients may have an annoying cough and may even have hemoptysis. On exam, a diastolic rumble can be heard along with an opening snap. Patients may also have a louder than normal S_1. Symptoms of CHF may be present with dyspnea, crackles, and rales heard in the lungs as well as fatigue. Atrial fibrillation may also be detected either palpably or on EKG. Symptoms are worse in females during pregnancy because of the increased blood volume that is present and the strain this puts on the mitral valve.

Conservative management is used to treat patients with mitral stenosis, but the valve can be replaced if there is no other option. Endocarditis prophylaxis is required.

Mitral insufficiency

Mitral insufficiency occurs when the mitral valve begins to degenerate. It can be due to rheumatic fever, congenital disorders, endocarditis, or myxoma cardiac tumors. Dysfunction of the papillary muscles can also lead to mitral insufficiency as can coronary artery disease.

The symptoms of mitral insufficiency may be acute of chronic. Patients may complain of shortness of breath with activity, fatigue, and weakness. A holosystolic murmur can be heard over the cardiac apex, and this murmur will radiate into the axilla area. An S_3 may also be heard. Patients may exhibit signs of CHF with rales, crackles, and dyspnea. Atrial fibrillation may be palpable or present on EKG. A chest x-ray and EKG can show the signs of CHF and left ventricular hypertrophy or cardiomegaly. Pulmonary edema may also be present. If due to papillary muscle dysfunction, patients may present in cardiogenic shock if a papillary muscle has ruptured. This is a life-threatening emergency with a very poor prognosis.

Mitral valve prolapse

Mitral valve prolapse is more common in females and is a condition in which the mitral valve leaflets are bulging into the atrium. It can be congenital in nature with Marfan's syndrome or connective tissue disorders, or may be due to CAD or cardiomyopathy. It is most likely due to congenital changes and is frequently seen in multiple members of a family.

Patients may complain of chest pain and shortness of breath with activity. They will be fatigued and may feel palpitations at times. They may also be completely asymptomatic. On exam, a midsystolic ejection click can be head with a mid to late systolic murmur.

Tricuspid stenosis

Stenosis of the tricuspid valve is frequently due to carcinoid tumors, rheumatic fever, or endocarditis. It is not very common and can result in right atrial enlargement. The right ventricle may appear smaller than normal because of the decreased amount of blood entering the chamber.

Patients with tricuspid stenosis may be fatigued and frequently feel cold. They may notice a fluttering sensation in the neck or palpitations. If the condition is advanced, they may feel abdominal pain and bloating due to hepatomegaly. On exam, symptoms of right-sided CHF may be seen, including pitting edema. A bounding pulse may be palpated in the neck over the carotid arteries. A diastolic rumble can be auscultated. Chest x-ray will show right atrial enlargement with right ventricular shrinkage. An echocardiogram can measure the amount of blood flow through the valves and determine if the flow through the tricuspid valve is decreased. Very rarely, the valve is damaged badly enough that surgery is required to repair or replace it.

Tricuspid insufficiency

Tricuspid insufficiency is more common than tricuspid stenosis. Each time the right ventricle contracts, there is blood flow backward through the tricuspid valve. It can occur due to muscle damage in the right ventricle from an acute MI. It may be due to right ventricular overload, endocarditis, or congenital anomalies. It can also occur due to mitral valve disease. A congenital condition called Ebstein's anomaly can result in an abnormally formed tricuspid valve, resulting in enlargement of the right atrium and congestive heart failure.

Patients may complain of swelling in their extremities that is not completely relieved with elevation. They may feel fatigued and have shortness of breath with activity. On exam, the symptoms of right-sided CHF may be seen with pulmonary edema and right atrial enlargement on chest x-ray. A harsh systolic murmur can be auscultated. If severe, there may be symptoms of hepatomegaly, and patients may complain of abdominal discomfort.

Pulmonary stenosis

Pulmonary stenosis is most often due to congenital abnormalities and is frequently seen along with other cardiac abnormalities. It can also occur as a result of rheumatic fever or endocarditis.

Patients may complain of fatigue and shortness of breath with activity. They may have episodes of chest pain, especially with activity, and may have even had syncopal episodes. They may have cyanosis due to decreased flow of blood to the lungs for oxygenation, though this is usually only present in very advanced stages. A mid-systolic murmur will be present that tends to increase with breathing. A wide split S_2 can be present with a right ventricular heave. Symptoms of right-sided CHF may be present with edema and right atrial enlargement on chest x-ray. Infants may exhibit failure to thrive and poor weight gain.

Surgery is often necessary to repair the valve. A valvuloplasty can be performed in children and adults, though not infants. Valvuloplasty involves stretching the valve with a balloon in order to widen the opening.

<u>Pulmonary insufficiency</u>
Pulmonary insufficiency can occur in patients who suffer from pulmonary hypertension. It can also be due to endocarditis, rheumatic heart disease, congenital abnormalities, or carcinoid syndrome.

Patients may complain of fatigue, chest pain, and shortness of breath with activity. There are usually no symptoms with this condition until it becomes advanced. Patients can have syncopal episodes if symptoms become severe. On exam, a low-pitched murmur, which may increase with breathing, may be heard. When pressure rises in the pulmonary artery with advanced disease, a Graham-Steel murmur, which is a high-pitched blowing decrescendo murmur, can be heard. There will be a widely split S_2, and a right-sided S_3 or S_4 may be heard during breathing. On EKG, right ventricular hypertrophy will be seen along with a right bundle branch block.

Usually the symptoms are not severe enough to warrant treatment with replacement of the pulmonary valve, but surgery can be done if patients are extremely symptomatic.

Endocarditis

A patient with heart disease affecting the valves is at risk for developing endocarditis. This includes those with congenital heart disease or valvular disease and those who have prosthetic valves. IV drug abusers and those who have had a prior infection are also at risk. Endocarditis can also be acquired through contamination during invasive procedures or surgery.

Almost all patients with endocarditis will have a new, regurgitant-type murmur. They may complain of fatigue. Splinter hemorrhages may be evident in the nail beds with Osler nodes and Janeway lesions present in the fingers. Roth spots may be evident on funduscopic exam and patients may show signs of emboli being present, such as hematuria and renal dysfunction. Anemia may be present with leukocytosis.

Appropriate antibiotic therapy based on culture and sensitivity results should be used for treatment. These patients will require prophylactic antibiotics for future invasive procedures. Treatment includes amoxicillin 2 g one hour before the procedure. If people have penicillin allergy, clindamycin 600 mg or azithromycin 500 mg is given one hour before the procedure.

<u>Diagnosis</u>

A patient must have 2 major criteria, 1 major and 3 minor criteria, or 5 minor criteria in order to be diagnosed with endocarditis. The major criteria are two positive blood cultures that indicate which organism is causing the infection and evidence of endocardial involvement on an echocardiogram or the presence of a new regurgitant murmur.

The minor criteria are risk factors, a fever >100.4°F, vascular features such as emboli, immunologic features such as glomerulonephritis, a positive blood culture that does not meet a major criteria, and changes on an echocardiogram that do not meet the major criteria.

The blood cultures should be drawn three times with the samples taken 1 hour apart. The most likely organism to cause endocarditis is *Streptococcus viridians* with *Staphylococcus aureus* the second most common. The echocardiogram will show vegetation on the valves in the heart, and a transesophageal echocardiogram may be necessary for accurate visualization.

Acute pericarditis

Acute pericarditis occurs when the pericardial sac becomes inflamed. This can most commonly be due to a viral infection, but a bacterial or parasitic infection can also cause this condition. Connective tissue disorders, such as lupus or rheumatoid arthritis, can also cause pericarditis, as can metabolic disorders such as renal failure and gout. Patients with pericarditis will complain of pleuritic chest pain that is relieved by sitting up and leaning forward. They will have a nonproductive cough accompanied with dyspnea. They will also have pain through the trapezius muscle, either unilaterally or bilaterally. On exam, a pericardial rub may be heard and leukocytosis may be present. An EKG will show ST elevation and PR depression. An echocardiogram will indicate a pericardial effusion.

Treatment is with NSAIDs, aspirin, and steroids to reduce the inflammation. If severe, a pericardial window may be created surgically to reduce the tension on the pericardial sac. In rare cases, the pericardial sac is completely removed to treat this condition.

Cardiac tamponade

Cardiac tamponade is an emergency condition in which fluid accumulates around the heart, leading to constriction that decreases venous return to the heart and prevents the ventricles from filling. It can occur with pericarditis, acute MI, a dissecting thoracic aortic aneurysm, or end-stage lung cancer. Patients who have undergone recent cardiac surgery are also at risk of developing a cardiac tamponade.

A *pulsus paradoxus*, which is a >10 mm drop in systolic pressure during inspiration, can be present. The pulse pressure will be narrowed, and patients will be hypotensive. Patients will be tachypneic, and jugular venous distention will be present. A Swan line to measure pressure within the heart will reveal that all of the pressures are equal.

Cardiac tamponade is diagnosed through echocardiogram and chest x-ray. It is an emergency situation, and an immediate pericardiocentesis should be performed to withdraw the fluid off the heart. It is often fatal.

Pericardial effusion

A pericardial effusion occurs when >250 cc of fluid accumulates within the pericardial space. It can occur due to a viral infection, tuberculosis, radiation to the chest cavity, or trauma. A malignant tumor in the chest cavity can also cause a pericardial effusion.

Patients with pericardial effusion do not always complain of chest pain. They will have a cough and appear dyspneic. If the cause is infection, they may have a fever. On exam, distant sounds with a pericardial rub will be heard.

Chest-x-ray will show cardiomegaly with a globular shape. EKG changes will be non-specific and may show a low voltage QRS complex. Treatment can include NSAIDs and steroids to treat the inflammation, but surgery frequently needs to be done to drain off the fluid. In severe cases, the pericardial sac can be completely removed from around the heart. A pericardial biopsy may also need to be done to determine the cause of the effusion.

Dermatologic

Atopic dermatitis

Atopic dermatitis, or eczema, is a skin rash that is more prevalent in children than adults though it can occur at any time in life. The exact cause is not known, but it is thought to be immune-mediated. It is frequently seen along with asthma or hay fever. Stress can exacerbate symptoms.

Patients will have reddish to dark-colored discolored areas on the skin and are extremely pruritic. This pruritus is worse at night and can be aggravated by temperature changes, hot showers or baths, or allergens such as cigarette smoke. Atopic dermatitis most often occurs over the antecubital fossa, behind the knees, and on the feet, though it can occur anywhere on the body. The areas may have small papules that can become fluid-filled and will crust over after opening.

Lubricating creams and oils can be used in infants with eczema. Topical corticosteroid creams can also be used when prescribed. Avoiding irritants that trigger the outbreaks also helps to decrease the symptoms.

Contact dermatitis

Contact dermatitis is an allergic response to an allergen. This can be caused by skin irritants, such as lotions and soaps or poison ivy and poison sumac. The skin rash associated with contact dermatitis often occurs quickly following exposure to the allergen.

Symptoms include an extremely pruritic rash. The skin will become red, and vesicular lesions that resemble a burn may be present. The skin can become red, dry, and cracked when exposed to irritants and may not develop the typical contact dermatitis lesions seen with exposure to an allergen.

Treatment requires discontinuing exposure to the causative substance. The skin should be kept clean and dry. Anti-itch medications or corticosteroid creams can be applied. Benadryl can be taken if the dermatitis is due to exposure to an allergen. This will help to decrease the release of histamine. If contact dermatitis is severe, oral steroids can be given to reduce the inflammation.

Diaper rash

Diaper rash is very common and occurs in babies wearing diapers or in adults who are incontinent. It is caused by exposure of the skin to the moisture of urine and waste material. If severe, the rash can develop into a bacterial or fungal infection.

The skin that has the moisture against it will become very inflamed and red. There may be areas where the skin is broken or cracked. The area will be very tender. If a fungal infection develops because of the moisture, there may be small red papules surrounding the inflamed area.

The goal of treating diaper rash is to keep the skin clean and dry. Leaving the skin open to air and avoiding a wet diaper against the skin will help to relieve the rash. Barrier creams and ointment containing zinc oxide can help to prevent further irritation of the skin. An antifungal or antibacterial cream may be necessary if a secondary infection occurs.

Nummular eczema

Nummular eczema is a form of eczema that causes coin-shaped patches on the skin. There is no definite known cause, but it does tend to be aggravated by strong soaps and detergents. Abrasive fabrics and extremes in temperature can also aggravate the condition.

The lesions with nummular eczema are initially often confused with a drug allergy. They are very pruritic and tend to be dry and scaly. The rash can also resemble a fungal infection or ringworm, but it tends to occasionally re-occur.

Treatment is with strong corticosteroid creams or ointments to help control the symptoms. With a severe outbreak, short-term oral steroids may be necessary. Coal tar preparations can help with an outbreak, but they tend to stain clothing. A secondary skin infection may develop with persistent itching of the skin, and appropriate antibiotic therapy should be given if this occurs.

Avoiding the triggers that cause flare-ups of the condition is necessary to decrease the severity and frequency of outbreaks.

Dyshidrosis

Dyshidrosis, or dyshidrotic eczema, is a form of eczema that causes vesicular lesions to form on the palms and soles. This condition is more common in women than men, and the exact cause is not known. It seems to occur more frequently during stressful times, and may be linked to exposure to metal salts. There also seems to be an increased incidence of this condition in those patients who suffer from hay fever.

Symptoms include extremely pruritic vesicular lesions on the palms of the hands and soles of the feet. These will break open and can crust over. As the lesions are resolving, the skin becomes very dry and cracked, and this can be painful. Secondary skin infections can occur when there are breaks in the skin.

Dyshidrosis is a chronic condition, and there is no known cure. Corticosteroid creams or ointments can help with symptoms, and antihistamines may decrease the severity of the flare-ups. UV light therapy can also help to control the symptoms during an outbreak.

Lichen planus

Lichen planus is a skin condition that appears to be immune-mediated. The exact cause is not known, but it may be linked to a drug allergy. Patients with hepatitis C have shown an increased incidence of this condition, but a definite link cannot be confirmed.

The lesions seen with lichen planus are flat-topped papules that usually form a row. It most commonly occurs around the ankles or the distal upper extremities. It can also become severe and form over the oral mucosa and the genitals, or any other part of the body. The lesions are very pruritic and may burn. Once the lesions fade, they may leave a darker pigmented scar on the skin.

Lichen planus usually resolves spontaneously within 1 year, but symptoms can be controlled with creams containing immunomodulating medications. If severe, oral steroids may be necessary. Antihistamines and UV light therapy may also be helpful in controlling the symptoms of lichen planus.

Stevens-Johnson syndrome

Stevens-Johnson syndrome, or erythema multiforme major, is a severe condition that usually occurs due to a medication reaction or illness. Antibiotics, NSAIDs, and anticonvulsant medications are most likely to cause this syndrome. Patients who are immunocompromised are more likely to develop this condition, and there may be a genetic link that causes some people to be more susceptible.

Patients will have vague, flu-type symptoms for a few days followed by development of an erythematous to purple rash over the oral mucous membranes. This can form vesicles and swelling and will spread over the skin. Eventually, the top-most layer of skin will slough off.

Hospitalization is necessary to treat Stevens-Johnson syndrome. Fluid replacement and wound care is needed, along with supportive therapy. If the syndrome is severe, immunoglobulin therapy may be necessary to control the symptoms. Skin grafting may be necessary if the skin loss is severe. It may take several months for patients to recover from this condition.

Folliculitis

Folliculitis is an infection around the hair follicle. It can be mild and self-limiting or may be reoccurring and painful. The most common causes are frequent shaving, perspiration in the area of the infection, and chronic inflammatory conditions of the skin. It can also be linked to exposure of the skin to coal tar or pitch.

Patients will have small erythematous pustules surrounding the hair. These pustules may break open and crust over. Lesions may be pruritic or tender. Folliculitis can occasionally involve a large area and cause swelling and extreme pain. Warm compresses can help relieve the symptoms, and folliculitis will usually resolve spontaneously without medical treatment after a few days. If severe, or caused by *Staphylococcus* or MRSA, antibiotics may be necessary to treat the condition. The most common causative organism is *Staphylococcus*. If patients have excessive exposure to water on their skin, *Pseudomonas* may be the cause.

Basal cell carcinoma

Basal cell carcinoma is the most common and slowest-growing form of skin cancer. It is caused by excessive exposure to UV light. Patients who develop a basal cell lesion are very likely to have more in the future.

The lesions with basal cell are usually pearly white to brown in color and may have a waxy appearance. They can be flat or scaly in appearance. These tend to bleed if picked at and will crust over and heal. There may be a depressed area in the center and superficial blood vessels may be visible on the lesion.

Treatment of basal cell carcinoma is with removal of the lesion. This can be surgically excised or removed with laser therapy, cryotherapy, or antineoplastic creams, such as 5-fluorouracil. Patients should be educated on the importance of protecting the skin from sun exposure. Sunscreen with a high SPF level should be used whenever patients are outside.

Melanoma

Melanoma is the most serious form of skin cancer and can be fatal. It develops in the melanin cells of the skin and can metastasize internally. It is more likely to occur in those who are fair skinned and those who have a positive family history of melanoma. It is caused by exposure to UV light.

Melanoma can develop in a mole or may be a new lesion on the skin. The discolored skin will have asymmetrical borders, and the color will change over time. The lesion may be flat or appear as a bump. Melanoma lesions are usually at least ¼-inch in diameter and may become hard or bumpy.

Treatment is with surgical excision to include a small amount of surrounding normal tissue. Diagnostic studies should be done to ensure there has not been any metastasis of the melanoma. Regular checks with a dermatologist and vigilant use of sunscreen are necessary. Skin should be shielded from the sun when outside.

Squamous cell carcinoma

Squamous cell carcinoma is a form of skin cancer that can spread to surrounding tissue, lymph nodes, and organs and can be fatal if left untreated. Though not as deadly as melanoma, squamous cell carcinoma is more likely to cause serious complications than basal cell carcinoma. Squamous cell carcinoma is caused by exposure to UV light and is more likely to occur in men than women, especially those who are fair-skinned. It is thought that smokers and those with human papilloma virus (HPV) infection are more likely to develop squamous cell lesions.

Squamous cell carcinoma lesions are usually red and firm. These can occur anywhere on the body and the appearance may vary. They can be crusty or scaly and may appear white when forming on mucous membranes.

Treatment is with removal of the lesion. This can be accomplished with excision, laser therapy, or cryotherapy. The skin should always be protected from sun by shielding or applying sunscreen with a high SPF rating.

Varicella-zoster infection

A varicella-zoster infection, or shingles, can be a very painful condition. It is caused by the same virus that causes chickenpox in children. The virus lies dormant in the nerve cells. Increased stress, an immunocompromised state, or other infections may cause the virus to be reactivated, resulting in shingles.

Patients will complain of burning pain at the site of the lesions and may develop this sensation before the lesions appear. Lesions most frequently occur around the chest wall, following a dermatomal pattern, though they can occur anywhere on the body, including the face and eyes. The vesicular lesions will open and eventually crust over. Patients may be left with chronic pain, called post-herpetic neuralgia, after the lesions resolve.

Treatment is with antivirals, such as acyclovir, to help decrease the length and severity of the outbreak. Topical anesthetics, such as Lidocaine patches, can also help to decrease the pain. Anticonvulsants and antidepressants may help with the lasting pain of post-herpetic neuralgia.

EENT (Eyes, Ears, Nose and Throat)

Blepharitis

Blepharitis is an inflammation or infection of the eyelid and eyelashes. There are two types, Staphylococcus *blepharitis* and *Seborrheic blepharitis*, with *seborrheic* being the most common. In addition to the eyelids and eyelashes, blepharitis can affect the eyebrows and scalp.

Patients may complain of burning of the eyes and matting of the eyelashes. The eyes may be irritated with a gritty feeling. They can also appear red.

Treating blepharitis involves debriding the lid margin of the matted material, usually using a cotton applicator. Warm compresses may be helpful and can be soothing to patients. Topical antibiotics may be given and should be applied in the morning and at bedtime to prevent blurred vision from interfering with daily activities. Antihistamine eye drops do not help to relieve the symptoms of blepharitis caused by *Seborrhea* or *Staphylococcus*. If the irritation is allergic in origin, then the drops will have an immediate effect. Lubricating eye drops will not help to relieve the gritty feeling patients experience.

Blowout fracture

A blowout fracture is a fracture of the orbital floor and involves the maxillary bone and the posterior medial floor of the orbit. It occurs due to excessive facial trauma.

These patients will report trauma and complain of significant pain. Diplopia may be present because of restriction of the extraocular muscles. The eyelid may be edematous with crepitus present on palpation. A potential complication of a blowout fracture is possible entrapment of the orbital contents within the maxillary sinus. If this occurs, the eye may have a sunken appearance, or enophthalmos.

A blowout fracture will typically heal on its own with regular follow-up to ensure proper healing is occurring. Patients should be advised to avoid blowing their noses. Oral antibiotics may be given to decrease the risk of orbital infection. In some cases, such as with restrictive diplopia or enophthalmos, surgery may be necessary to repair the orbital wall.

Chalazion

A chalazion is caused by the inflammation of a sebaceous gland on the eyelid. It is not the same thing as a sty. A sty will also involve hair follicles and is more superficial appearing.

A chalazion usually occurs on the upper eyelid. There may be gradual swelling that increases over the course of a few days to a few weeks. The lesion may appear red and inflamed, and patients may complain of pain.

Warm compresses may help to relieve the pain and promote absorption of the oil that is trapped in the sebaceous gland. If a bacterial infection is superimposed on the chalazion, an ophthalmic antibiotic may be prescribed. An injection of triamcinolone (Kenalog®) directly into the mass may help to relieve the inflammation and promote healing. In rare cases, surgical incision of the mass may be necessary if it persists and is not resolving with more conservative treatments.

Conjunctivitis

Conjunctivitis ("pink eye") is an infection of the conjunctiva of one or both eyes. It can be caused by a bacteria or virus or can be allergic in nature.

Patients will complain of a gritty, irritating, itching sensation in the eye, which is red from hemorrhage of small vessels. Vision is usually not affected. With bacterial conjunctivitis, there is a mucus discharge, and patients may have problems with the eye being matted closed in the morning. Viral and allergic conjunctivitis typically cause a watery discharge.

If bacterial conjunctivitis is suspected, ophthalmic antibiotics to treat *Staphylococcus* or *Streptococcus* infection should be given to adults. If severe, *Gonococcal* conjunctivitis, which will require IV antibiotics, should be considered. In children, *Staphylococcus* or *Streptococcus* can cause the infection, as well as *Haemophilus*. Viral conjunctivitis only requires symptomatic relief. Patients should avoid rubbing the eye. Frequent hand washing can decrease transmission of the condition.

Allergic conjunctivitis can be treated with ophthalmic antihistamines, but this condition may be chronic in patients who suffer from recurrent environmental allergies.

Corneal abrasion

A corneal abrasion is caused by minor trauma to the surface of the eye, resulting in a scratching of the cornea. Patients will complain of pain and tearing of the eye, and may even complain of blurred vision.

To diagnose a corneal abrasion, topical anesthetics should be instilled in the eye. Fluorescein is then administered in the eye, and an ultraviolet light is used to examine the eye. The area of the cornea that is affected will brightly light up, indicating the area of abrasion. The eye should be gently irrigated to ensure there are no lingering foreign objects that can continue to cause damage. Topical anti-inflammatory drugs can be prescribed to help with pain relief and topical antibiotics may or may not be given to prevent the development of infection. Depending on patients' discomfort level, the eye can be patched for a couple of days to prevent further irritation. This condition should heal within a couple of days of treatment.

Dacryocystitis

Dacryocystitis is a condition in which the lacrimal sac becomes inflamed. This inflammation can be due to a blockage at some point in the tear drainage system or a stone that has formed within the lacrimal sac.

Patients will complain of pain along the inside corner of the eye. The area will appear red and swollen and may extend from the inner canthus of the eye to the upper nose or nasal bridge.

To treat this inflammation and infection, antibiotics can be given. Depending upon the severity, patients may require hospitalization for IV antibiotic therapy. If severe, incision and drainage may be necessary to treat an abscess. Once the inflammation and infection have resolved, surgery may be necessary to correct the blockage. If a stone is present within the lacrimal sac, this will need to be surgically removed to prevent future blockages leading to abscess formation.

Ectropion and entropion

An ectropion is a condition in which the lower eyelid turns outward. This usually occurs during the aging process due to laxity of the muscles within the eyelid. The ectropion causes dryness and irritation of the eye. A paralysis of the facial nerve can cause this to occur because of the loss of neuromuscular control of the facial muscles on the affected side. Scarring due to trauma or burns can also cause an ectropion. Repair of the ectropion is accomplished through surgery to tighten the muscles of the lower eyelid.

An entropion is a condition in which the lower eyelid turns inward. This is most commonly caused by the aging process due to muscle laxity causing the lower eyelid to involute. Facial nerve palsy and scarring can also cause this condition. Patients will complain of irritation of the eye with tearing and the sensation of a foreign body being in the eye due to the eyelashes rubbing on the sclera. Treatment is by surgical correction.

Glaucoma

To diagnose glaucoma, the angle at which fluid flows from the eye is measured. The pressure is measured within the eye to determine if it is increased. With primary open angle glaucoma, the angle is open with the presence of optic nerve damage and a loss of peripheral vision found on visual field testing. It is the most common form of glaucoma and is usually age-related.

Treatment begins with ophthalmic eye drops. Ophthalmic beta-blockers, such as Timolol, can be used. Medications such as Pilocarpine that work on the muscarinic receptors of the eye to increase fluid flow are also prescribed. There has been some controversy over whether to start with medical treatment or proceed with surgical treatment first for primary open angle glaucoma. Laser treatment and traditional surgical treatment are usually reserved for treatment once medical management has failed to produce adequate results in decreasing the ocular pressure.

Angle closure glaucoma

There are two types of angle closure glaucoma: primary and acute.

Primary angle closure glaucoma affects approximately 10% of those patients who have glaucoma. The angle through which fluid drains from the eye is narrowed, resulting in an increase in ocular pressure. This is treated with surgery by creating an opening behind the iris through which the fluid can flow from the eye, resulting in a decrease in ocular pressure.

Acute angle closure glaucoma results in the sudden onset of blurred vision with visual halos, pain, red eye, and possibly nausea and vomiting. This requires urgent treatment. The cornea may be edematous when examined, and ocular pressure readings are extremely elevated with this condition. Medications may be necessary at first to reduce the corneal edema. Ultimately, laser surgery is necessary to open the angle so that fluid can flow from the eye to cause a decrease in the ocular pressure.

Hordeolum

A hordeolum, or "stye," is a condition in which an eyelash follicle becomes infected. Patients may complain of tenderness around the area. The small abscess will appear red and swollen. It will eventually come to a head and purulent discharge may be expressed from the small infection.

Treatment of a hordeolum generally consists of frequent application of warm compresses to draw the abscess to a head so that the infectious material can be expressed. The hordeolum may not drain and can resolve on its own. If the condition becomes severe, or if patients develop recurrent hordeola, tetracycline may be given to eradicate the infection. It is important to remember that children should not be given tetracycline because of alterations that can occur in tooth or bone development. Tetracycline should also not be given to females who are or may become pregnant because of the risk of birth anomalies.

Hyphema

Hyphema is blood in the anterior chamber of the eye. It is most frequently caused by blunt trauma to the eye, but can also occur following eye surgery or certain medical disorders, such as sickle cell anemia. A hyphema is very obvious because blood will be visible underneath the cornea and cause the iris to be blocked. There may also be conjunctival hemorrhages present.

Treatment involves strict activity restrictions with avoidance of all strenuous activities. Aspirin and other anticoagulant medications should be avoided to decrease the risk of additional bleeding. If the hyphema is managed on an outpatient basis, patients should be re-evaluated every couple of days to assess for rebleeding. Bleeding can reoccur 3-6 days following the initial eye trauma and may be worse than the initial bleeding that caused the hyphema. Once the hyphema has resolved, patients should continue to be evaluated annually because these patients are at risk for developing glaucoma later in life.

Macular degeneration

Macular degeneration is the most common cause of blindness in the Caucasian population. It is rare in other races. There are two types of macular degeneration: dry and wet.

The dry form is more common and occurs when drusen are deposited deep in the eye near the retina. It begins in middle age and progresses slowly, causing a loss of central vision not usually resulting in legal blindness. It can, however, develop into wet macular degeneration.

Wet macular degeneration occurs when capillaries break through the retina and grow behind the macula of the eye. This form of the disease is more debilitating and can lead to legal blindness.

There is no definitive cure for macular degeneration. Vitamins A, D, and E slow the progress of dry macular degeneration. Medications (Lucentis®, Macugen®, and Visudyne®) and surgery may improve vision in wet macular degeneration. There is a genetic link with this disease and prevention is key. Eating leafy green vegetables high in carotenoids, quitting smoking, and protecting the eyes from UV light, can reduce risk.

Orbital cellulitis

Orbital cellulitis is an infection that results in cellulitis of the eyelids. It is a serious condition and must be managed urgently to prevent further complications. Patients will have a painfully swollen and red eye, sometimes severe enough to cause the eye to be swollen shut. Patients may have blurred or double vision along with a headache. They may be febrile if the infection is severe. On exam, the eye may be displaced anteriorly with a sluggish pupil reaction to light. The extraocular movements may also be restricted, depending on the amount of edema. A CT scan can be done to rule out the presence of a foreign body and to assess any damage to the optic nerve.

Patients usually require hospitalization and treatment with IV antibiotics. *Staphylococcus* is the most common cause of bacterial infection, but immunocompromised patients may develop a fungal orbital cellulitis. Once the infection is controlled with IV antibiotics, patients can be discharged home on oral antibiotics with close follow-up.

Pterygium

A pterygium is a triangular-shaped raised lesion that grows on the surface of the eye. It most commonly occurs on the nasal side of the cornea and may appear red. Patients usually seek treatment for this because of cosmetic appearances, but it can grow to obstruct the visual fields. This occurs if it extends over the cornea. Occasionally, it can be irritating to the eye.

Treatment involves surgical removal of the pterygium, though this is usually reserved for cases in which the lesion affects the visual fields or is irritating. Surgery may be necessary to replace a portion of the conjunctiva. An antimetabolite may also be applied during surgery to prevent recurrence of the lesion. Almost one-half of patients who develop a pterygium will go on to develop the lesion again. There are usually no long-term effects of decreased visual acuity following surgery if the lesion is not encroaching upon the cornea.

Rhegmatogenous retinal detachment

Rhegmatogenous is the most common form of retinal detachment. Rhegmatogenous retinal detachment occurs when there is a tear in the retina, allowing the vitreous humor to enter the space behind the retina and causing a detachment of the retina from the posterior eye. The most common cause of this type of retinal detachment is the aging process, which leads to shrinkage of the vitreous humor. This causes pulling on the retina, leading to a tear or hole in the retina.

Patients will describe floaters and flashes of light with an associated decrease in vision. The loss of vision will occur in a curtain-type fashion, where the vision seems to be blocked out momentarily and then returns. This occurs as the torn retina flaps down and then back up. This condition is a surgical emergency and needs to be treated immediately. Delay of even one day can result in some degree of permanent visual loss after surgical repair.

Tractional retinal detachment

A tractional retinal detachment occurs in conditions that cause scarring within the vitreous humor, such as diabetic retinopathy. The fibrous strands that make up a scar cause traction to be applied to the retina. This traction results in separation of the retina from the posterior eye. Some patients may have floaters or flashes of light in their vision, along with the curtain-type vision loss, as seen with rhegmatogenous retinal detachment. More commonly, there will be visual loss with a description of blind spots in the vision.

Treatment of a tractional retinal detachment usually involves removing the vitreous humor, thereby removing the fibrous scar material. Gas or an oily substance may be injected into the eye to prevent recurrence of this condition. There is a chance of permanent visual loss with this condition, despite aggressive treatment. The best treatment is prevention by maintaining adequate control of blood sugar levels in diabetics to prevent the development of diabetic retinopathy.

Exudative retinal detachment

An exudative retinal detachment occurs when fluid builds up behind the retina. This can occur with several medical conditions, including various collagen-vascular diseases, posterior scleritis, tumors affecting the eye, and congenital abnormalities. This results in visual loss with patients complaining of experiencing blind spots in their vision. They may also experience floaters or flashes of light in their vision.

Surgery is not usually necessary to treat this condition. Treatment of the underlying condition is usually sufficient to prevent permanent visual loss. With chronic medical conditions that cause an exudative retinal detachment, achieving adequate medical control of the condition can result in reversal of the detachment as the fluid behind the retina dissipates. Urgent treatment of the cause of the retinal detachment is necessary to prevent permanent visual loss. Some patients may develop a chronic problem with this condition, and then surgery to prevent fluid accumulation behind the retina is necessary.

Hypertensive retinopathy

Uncontrolled blood pressure is the cause of hypertensive retinopathy. As pressure rises within the body's arteries, the small arteries in the eye are also affected. This results in narrowing of the retinal arteries and a decrease in blood flow to the structures of the eye. Patients may or may not notice a decrease in their visual acuity. On exam, narrowed retinal arteries are visible, along with retinal hemorrhages and possibly some swelling. A swollen optic nerve can result with malignant hypertension, a condition in which the diastolic blood pressure is >120 mm Hg.

Treatment of hypertensive retinopathy involves controlling the blood pressure with diet, exercise, and medications. Malignant hypertension is an emergency condition and should be treated immediately. This involves slowly decreasing the blood pressure, over several hours, with low doses of antihypertensive medications. Visual loss that results from hypertensive retinopathy may be permanent, but control of the blood pressure can prevent additional damage.

Diabetic retinopathy

Diabetic retinopathy is the leading cause of blindness in the US in diabetics <65-years-old. It begins as tiny microaneurysms in the retina. Exudates form in the retina as these aneurysms rupture. Patients frequently have no visual loss at this stage.

As retinopathy progresses, the exudates become larger and the rupturing aneurysms can lead to swelling of the macula. Patients may or may not have a decrease in visual acuity. Focal laser photocoagulation is done at this stage to decrease the macular edema by cauterizing the leaking microaneurysms.

The final stages of diabetic retinopathy occur when new vessels are developed around the optic nerve. These vessels are very fragile and are easily ruptured, which leads to bleeding within the retina and vitreous humor. As scar tissue forms, the fibrous strands of the scar may cause a tractional retinal detachment. Focal laser photocoagulation can be performed to decrease the rupture of these new vessels, but visual loss is common with this condition, and blindness frequently occurs.

Strabismus

Strabismus is a condition in which the extraocular muscles are weakened, leading to a gaze deviation in one eye. It differs from a "lazy eye," or amblyopia, because there is no loss of visual acuity associated with a strabismus.

The condition is labeled by the direction in which the gaze is affected:

- Hypertropia occurs when the gaze is diverted upward.
- Exotropia when the gaze is deviated outward.
- Esotropia when the gaze is deviated inward ("cross-eyes").
- Hypotropia when the gaze is deviated downward.

A wide, flattened nose with a skin fold at the inner canthus can cause the appearance of esotropia and is called pseudoesotropia. This usually resolves with age. Eye muscle strengthening can be performed to help straighten the gaze in mild cases of strabismus. If this fails or if the strabismus is severe, surgery may be necessary to draw the affected muscles tighter in order to straighten the gaze.

Otitis media

Otitis media is an infection of the middle ear. It is most commonly bacterial or viral and affects children more often than adults because of the straight anatomic structure of the auditory canal and eustachian tube, which promotes the accumulation of fluid behind the tympanic membrane.

The most common cause of otitis media in children is infection with *Streptococcus, Pneumoniae,* or *H. influenzae*. The incidence of infection with these organisms is on the decline, however, because of immunizations now available to help prevent infection. *M. catarrhalis* can also cause otitis media. In immunocompromised individuals, fungal infections can lead to otitis media.

Symptoms include ear pain and fever. Symptoms of an upper respiratory infection may also be present. On exam, a bulging tympanic membrane with purulent effusion may be evident. There should be decreased movement of the membrane with insufflation.

Treatment is with oral antibiotics that will treat the most causative organisms. Drug resistance varies across the US, so current guidelines for any specific area should be followed.

Labyrinthitis

Labyrinthitis is an inflammatory condition affecting the labyrinth of the inner ear. It usually occurs following a viral infection, such as a cold or the flu. Bacterial infections of the upper respiratory system can also cause labyrinthitis. Trauma to the head or ear, along with benign tumors of the ear, can also cause this condition.

Vertigo is the main symptom that patients will experience. This can be quite severe with nausea and vomiting, along with a complete loss of balance. Patients may have a headache and may experience tinnitus with the condition. The symptoms can be positional or may occur at rest.

Labyrinthitis is usually treated with anti-vertigo medications, such as Antivert®. Rarely, antibiotics will be given if it is suspected the condition is caused by a bacterial infection. Small stones within the labyrinth can occasionally cause this condition, and the Epley maneuver can be used to change the position of the stones.

Otitis externa

Otitis externa is an infection of the external ear canal. It is usually caused by *Pseudomonas* bacteria, but can also be due to *Staphylococcus* or *Streptococcus* infections. Rarely, the infection can be due to a fungal infection. This is often referred to as "swimmer's ear" because of the prevalence in those who spend a lot of time in the water.

Patients will complain of significant ear pain that is exacerbated with movement of the external ear. Patients may or may not have enlargement of the preauricular lymph nodes. Exam of the ear canal will reveal edema and erythema of the ear canal, possibly with some purulent discharge.

A wick is placed in the ear canal to facilitate installation of an acidic solution. This will cure the otitis externa within a few days. Aminoglycoside eardrops can also be used, but care should be taken to ensure the tympanic membrane is intact because of the risk of ototoxicity with these medications. A topical fluoroquinolone is preferred over the aminoglycosides.

Mastoiditis

Mastoiditis is an infection of the mastoid bone of the skull and usually occurs following otitis media. In the past, mastoiditis was relatively common and the leading common cause of death in children. Since the advent of antibiotics and prompt treatment of otitis media infections, the incidence of mastoiditis has greatly declined.

Patients, if old enough, may complain of severe pain in the ear and behind the ear. There may be swelling in the area that causes the affected ear to stick out from the head. Patients may have a high fever and headache. A skull x-ray or CT of the head will show a honeycomb appearance of the mastoid bone due to the infection.

Treatment is with aggressive IV antibiotics in order to penetrate the bone tissue and treat the infection. If IV antibiotics are effective, patients will continue on oral antibiotics to completely eradicate the infection. If medical treatment is not effective, incision and drainage of the bone may be necessary to drain the infection.

Ménière's disease

Ménière's disease is a condition affecting the labyrinth of the ear. The labyrinth is made up of bony and membranous portions. The membranous portion contains a fluid called endolymph. It is thought that Ménière's disease results when the membranous portion of the labyrinth ruptures, causing the endolymph to mix with perilymph, a fluid separating the membranous portion from the bony portion.

The symptoms of Ménière's disease include tinnitus, vertigo, and loss of hearing. Some patients experience a feeling of pressure within the affected ear(s). These symptoms are often not constant, but rather occur intermittently.

There is no cure of Ménière's disease. The symptoms can be decreased, though, with the dietary restriction of sodium, caffeine, and alcohol. Quitting smoking may help decrease the severity of symptoms. Gentamycin eardrops may help decrease the vertigo. With severe cases, the labyrinth can be surgically removed, but this will result in a loss of hearing in the ear.

Sinusitis

Sinusitis usually occurs after a cold. The virus causing the cold results in swollen sinuses with increased mucus discharge. The mucus cannot drain because of the edematous sinuses, producing an excellent environment in which bacteria can thrive, leading to a sinus infection.

Patients will complain of cold symptoms that are present or resolving. They will have a headache, generally over the frontal, ethmoid, or maxillary sinuses. They may complain of positional increases in the headache and a full feeling or pressure within the head. A stuffy nose, fever, and aching in the teeth may also be present.

Treatment of sinusitis is with oral antibiotics. Drug resistance varies across the US, so appropriate treatment should be chosen depending on the area of the country. Decongestants may be helpful to promote drainage from the sinuses. Antipyretics and anti-inflammatory drugs can help with fever and headache pain.

Allergic rhinitis

Allergic rhinitis affects the nose and eyes. It occurs in those individuals with allergies to environmental irritants, such as pollen, animal dander, trees, and dust. The symptoms due to exposure from these irritants can vary from minor symptoms to hives and throat constriction.

The onset of symptoms can usually be associated with exposure to an environmental irritant. Symptoms include runny nose, itchy and watery eyes, mild cough, sneezing, facial itching, and sore throat. Patients may complain of a headache, possibly over the sinuses, with a feeling of pressure in the head. This is due to increased mucus production through the sinuses and nasal passages.

Antibiotics should not be used to treat the symptoms of allergic rhinitis. Antibiotics would only be used if there were a concomitant bacterial infection, such as sinusitis. Antihistamines can be given to decrease the release of histamine and suppress the allergic symptoms. Avoidance of the irritants is necessary to prevent symptoms. Nasal corticosteroid sprays can also help to decrease symptoms.

Pharyngitis

Pharyngitis is an inflammation of the pharynx, causing a sore throat. It is most commonly caused by a viral infection, such as the virus that causes the common cold. The most common bacterial cause of pharyngitis is Group A *Streptococcus.*

Patients will complain of a very sore throat that may or may not have been accompanied with other cold symptoms. Cold symptoms are usually present with viral forms of pharyngitis. A fever and headache may also be present. Children with *Streptococcal* pharyngitis may have some nausea and vomiting with the illness. On exam, cervical and tonsillar lymph nodes will be enlarged. The oropharynx will appear edematous and erythematous, possibly with white exudates present over the mucous membrane. A Quick Strep swabbing can be performed in the office to diagnose *streptococcal* pharyngitis, but definitive diagnosis is with culture and sensitivity of the causative organism.

Treatment of viral pharyngitis is supportive with warm salt water, antipyretics, and analgesics. Bacterial pharyngitis is treated with appropriate antibiotic therapy.

Aphthous ulcers

Aphthous ulcers, or canker sores, occur within the oral cavity. They can appear on the lips, oral mucosa, gums, or tongue. Canker sores are not contagious and always occur on the soft tissues of the mouth. They have no definite known cause, but irritants in the oral cavity, such as strongly acidic foods or candies, may contribute to aphthous ulcers.

Patients will complain of a painful area in the oral cavity with some swelling in the area. Exam will reveal a shallow, white or yellowish ulcer, usually less than 1 cm in width. There is usually no bleeding noticed, but there may be some edema and erythema of the surrounding tissue present.

Treatment of the ulcers involves avoiding acidic foods and drinks that irritate the ulcer. Smoking can also irritate the ulcer, as can very rough foods. Warm salt-water swish and swallow may be soothing to the lesion. Over-the-counter topical numbing medications may be helpful in decreasing the pain. Aphthous ulcers generally resolve spontaneously within a few days.

Dental abscess

A dental abscess is an infection that forms around the roots of a tooth, or teeth, or in the gum tissue. Infection within the dental pulp is more common in children while an abscess in the surrounding tissue is more common in adults.

Patients will develop severe pain in an isolated area of the mouth. The check will appear red and swollen, and lymph nodes in the neck on the affected side will be enlarged. A fever may be present as well as a headache. The abscess may rupture, resulting in a sudden rush of warm, foul-tasting and foul-smelling fluid in the mouth. The pain will subside after the abscess ruptures, but treatment is still necessary.

Treatment includes drainage of the abscess if it has not drained on its own. Antibiotics will be given to eradicate the infection after drainage. Antibiotic treatment of this infection is very important to prevent spread of the infection systemically.

Oral candidiasis

Oral candidiasis, or oral thrush, is a fungal infection affecting the oral mucosa. It is not contagious. It commonly occurs in those who wear dentures. It can also occur in diabetics, patients who take steroids (especially inhalation steroids), immunocompromised patients, and those taking antibiotics that affect the natural flora of the mouth. Radiation to the head and neck can also cause thrush.

Patients will have white plaques over the oral mucosa. The plaques can be scraped off with a tongue depressor to reveal red, raw areas. The lesions may or may not be painful to patients. Foul-smelling breath and alteration in taste are also common symptoms.

An antifungal swish and swallow solution is used to treat oral candidiasis. Impregnated swabs can also be used in those who are unable to swish the solution in their mouth before swallowing. Patients should be reminded to clean their dentures thoroughly daily. Patients using inhaled steroids should completely rinse their mouths after each treatment.

Oral leukoplakia

Oral leukoplakia is a white patchy lesion found in the oral cavity. It is caused by tobacco use, either smoking or chewing, and is considered a premalignant form of oral cancer. Another form of the condition is hairy leukoplakia, which is seen in HIV-positive patients or others with suppressed immune systems and is probably caused by the Epstein-Barr virus.

Patients will complain of a white patch in their mouths. This patch can be on the oral mucosa, the tongue, or gums. It is a painless, slightly raised, rough patch that is white or grayish in color. There may occasionally be leukoplakia lesions that appear pink or red in color. Eventually the lesion can become painful or sensitive to heat, cold, or spicy foods.

Treatment of oral leukoplakia is accomplished with surgical excision of the lesion. There is a chance that patients can develop these lesions again, especially if they continue to smoke or use smokeless tobacco. Quitting smoking is the best treatment for prevention of future lesions.

Peritonsillar abscess

A peritonsillar abscess can occur as a complication of bacterial tonsillitis. The causative organism is usually grouping A-beta hemolytic *Streptococcus*, but this condition is not as common as it was in the past because of the use of antibiotics to treat tonsillitis. An abscess can develop in the soft tissue surrounding the tonsil and lead to a severe infection.

Patients will have severe throat pain with enlarged lymph nodes on the affected side. They may have a fever and headache. There will be great difficulty swallowing, if they can swallow at all, and breathing may become compromised if the swelling is severe. Patients may have difficulty closing their mouths, and drooling may be evident.

The abscess should be drained, and culture and sensitivity testing should be done on the extracted pus. Treatment is with appropriate antibiotic therapy, and patients may require future surgery to remove the tonsils and prevent recurrence of this infection.

Parotitis

Parotitis, or mumps as it is more commonly known, is an infection of the salivary glands. It generally affects the parotid salivary glands, which are the largest. Mumps is a viral infection that is transmitted through airborne respiratory particles. It generally affects children more than adults, but there is an immunization available to prevent contraction of the disease.

Patients may complain of facial pain with a fever and headache. The affected side of the face will appear swollen, like "chipmunk cheeks." Parotitis can become systemic and affect the testes in boys and may lead to infertility.

Treatment is supportive. Because this is a viral illness, no antibiotic therapy is necessary. Ice or heat applied to the cheeks may help with pain relief, as can acetaminophen or ibuprofen for pain and fever relief. Chewing may be painful, so soft foods should be given with plenty of fluids. Boys should be frequently assessed for the formation of a lump or mass in the scrotum.

Sialadenitis

Sialadenitis is an infection of the salivary glands. It differs from parotitis, or mumps, in that it involves a blockage of the flow of saliva, causing bacteria to grow within the ducts. This leads to a bacterial infection, usually caused by *Staphylococcus aureus*. The most common salivary glands affected are the parotid gland in the cheek and the submandibular gland under the chin.

Patients will complain of pain in the affected area. Purulent drainage may flow into the mouth, causing a foul-smelling and foul-tasting sensation. Patients may have a fever and headache.

Treatment is usually accomplished with appropriate antibiotic therapy. If infection is severe, the gland may need to be drained with culture and sensitivity testing performed on the extracted pus. If a stone is causing a blockage of the ductwork leading from the salivary gland, this will need to be surgically removed. Patients may develop a chronic form of sialadenitis that causes recurrent flare-ups of the condition.

Endocrine

Parathyroid hormone

Parathyroid hormone, or PTH, is secreted by the parathyroid glands, which set posterior to the thyroid gland. Release of PTH is controlled by the pituitary gland's secretion of parathyroid stimulating hormone. The function of PTH is to control the body's calcium and phosphorus balance. When the calcium levels are low, PTH secretion is increased; when calcium levels rise, PTH secretion is suppressed. PTH causes calcium to be released from bones into the circulating blood stream.

Most commonly, an adenoma on the parathyroid glands can cause increased amounts of PTH to be released. With some types of cancer, there can be ectopic sources of parathyroid tissue that will secrete excess PTH. Multiple endocrine neoplasia syndromes can affect multiple endocrine glands, including the parathyroids, and lead to hyperparathyroidism. Accidental removal of the parathyroid glands during thyroid surgery can cause hypoparathyroidism. Hypomagnesemia can also cause there to be a decreased amount of PTH secreted by the glands. Rarely, there can be genetic causes of deficiencies in PTH secretion.

Hyperparathyroidism and hypoparathyroidism

Most patients with calcium levels <12 are asymptomatic. Symptoms usually begin as the calcium level rises above 12, and the symptoms will worsen as the calcium level continues to rise. Initially, patients may complain of nausea and vomiting with a loss of appetite. They may feel muscle weakness and fatigue. Constipation may be present. As the calcium level rises, they may become confused and lethargic. Polyuria can occur with renal failure. Cardiac arrhythmias can occur and even coma.

As calcium levels drop, patients may become confused or lethargic with mental status changes. Muscular changes with hypoparathyroidism will be the opposite of those with hyperparathyroidism. Patients will show signs of neuromuscular irritability with carpopedal spasm, laryngeal spasm, and facial grimacing. A positive Chvostek's sign, which will involve unilateral spasm of the facial muscles when the facial nerve is tapped, may be present. Patients may have seizures or cardiac arrhythmias when calcium levels are dangerously low.

Subacute thyroiditis

Most commonly, subacute thyroiditis is caused by a viral infection with coxsackie, mumps, influenza, or adenovirus. Patients will have a painful, tender, asymmetrically enlarged thyroid gland. They may remember having symptoms of an upper respiratory infection before the thyroid symptoms began. In addition to the localized tenderness, patients may describe symptoms of either hyper- or hypothyroidism. Usually, patients are initially in a hyperthyroid state, followed by a period of hypothyroidism, and then returning to a euthyroid state.

Lab tests will show an elevated WBC and sedimentation rate. Thyroid antibodies will be negative with this condition because it is not immune-mediated.

Patients are treated with NSAIDs, aspirin, or steroids to decrease the inflammation within the thyroid gland. Antibiotics do not have a role here because of the condition's viral etiology. The TSH and T4 levels should be monitored for resolution of subacute thyroiditis as this can take several months.

Cushing's syndrome

Cushing's syndrome results when cortisol levels are increased. Most commonly, this is due to steroid treatment with prednisone. A pituitary adenoma that causes excess amounts of adrenocorticotropic hormone (ACTH) will lead to elevated cortisol. A primary tumor of the adrenal gland may cause Cushing's due to increased cortisol secretion. Other forms of cancer can present with ectopic sources of ACTH secretion.

Patients will develop proximal muscle weakness and atrophy with an obtunded abdomen. Purple striae will develop across the abdomen. The face will be rounded ("moon face"), and fat deposition can occur across the upper back ("buffalo hump"). Patients will bruise easily and may have non-healing sores. Osteoporosis can occur, as can pathologic fractures. Glucose levels can be elevated, and patients may require insulin.

Primary treatment of Cushing's is to treat the cause. Patients should be weaned off prednisone if possible. Removal of a pituitary adenoma can decrease ACTH production. Removal of an adrenal adenoma or other ectopic source of hormone secretion can decrease cortisol levels.

Graves' disease

Graves' disease is a form of hyperthyroidism. It differs from hyperthyroidism in that exophthalmos and pretibial myxedema are usually present with Graves' disease whereas these two symptoms are not seen with regular hyperthyroidism. Along with those symptoms, patients may complain of irritability and nervousness, heat intolerance with increased sweating, and weight loss with an increase in appetite. Patients may be tachycardic and hypertensive and atrial fibrillation is not uncommon, especially in elderly patients. Hyperreflexia may be present and patients may have a fine tremor. Alopecia may occur, or the hair may be finer in texture. A goiter may be evident.

The cardiac symptoms of Graves' disease can be treated with beta-blockers. To control the thyroid gland, propylthiouracil (PTU) may be given. This can take 6-8 weeks to be effective. Radioactive iodine can also be given but takes approximately 2-3 months to normalize the thyroid. With iodine treatments, patients may convert to a hypothyroid state after several years.

Hashimoto's thyroiditis

Hashimoto's thyroiditis is an autoimmune-mediated form of hypothyroidism. The body's immune system attacks the thyroid tissue, preventing the normal secretion of thyroid hormones.

Patients may complain of symptoms of hypothyroidism, including fatigue, cold intolerance, weight gain with a decreased appetite, forgetfulness, dry skin, and a puffy face. Patients may or may not have a goiter. Female patients may also have increased menstrual flow.

Thyroid hormone levels may be normal early in the disease. The TSH level will be elevated, though, and the thyroid hormone levels will begin to decrease as the disease progresses. Anti-thyroid antibodies can also be tested to determine if this is autoimmune in etiology.

Treatment of Hashimoto's thyroiditis is accomplished through thyroid replacement hormone therapy. Blood tests are regularly performed to measure the thyroid hormone levels and ensure that patients have reached a therapeutic dose of hormone replacement therapy. Treatment should be continued through pregnancy.

Thyroid storm

A thyroid storm is very rare, but can be life-threatening. It is a situation in which the thyroid secretes a massive amount of thyroid hormones at one time, causing an acute state of hyperthyroidism. This can be due to a tumor, excessive manipulation during surgery, or trauma. Infections can increase thyroid hormone production. Patients who take excessive doses of thyroid hormone can also have symptoms of thyroid storm.

This can cause patients to develop CHF, cardiac arrhythmias, or hyperthermia. On a milder level, patients may develop a fever, vomiting and diarrhea, or disorientation and delirium. This can progress to the point of seizures or coma.

Beta-blockers should be given to treat the cardiac symptoms associated with a thyroid storm. Antiarrhythmic medications may be necessary if an arrhythmia develops. PTU can be given intravenously to suppress the secretion of thyroid hormones. Potassium iodide can also be given for this same purpose. Corticosteroids may be necessary to control any acute inflammation within the thyroid gland.

Hypothyroidism

Hypothyroidism is most commonly due to autoimmune factors, such as with Hashimoto's thyroiditis. Outside the US, a primary iodine deficiency is the most common cause of hypothyroidism. Pituitary tumors can also cause a decrease in TSH secretion, which will lead to secondary hypothyroidism. Patients may complain of fatigue and weakness with weight gain and a decreased appetite. The skin may be dry and coarse and patients may have edema of the face, hands, and feet (myxedema). There will be cold intolerance and a hoarse voice, hypertension and bradycardia, and reduced concentration and memory. Patients may describe paresthesias in the hands in a median nerve distribution.

Lab results with hypothyroidism will show an elevated TSH as the pituitary gland tries to stimulate more production of the thyroid hormones. T3 and T4, the primary thyroid hormones, will be decreased. With Hashimoto's thyroiditis, thyroid antibodies will be present.

Treatment is with thyroid replacement hormone and careful monitoring of the thyroid hormone levels to reach therapeutic dosage.

Adrenal insufficiency

Adrenal insufficiency can be primary or secondary. Primary, or Addison's disease, is due to autoimmune factors, infections, or disease within the adrenal gland. This causes a decrease in cortisol secretion. Secondary factors include a pituitary adenoma or acute discontinuation of steroid use.

Patients may complain of fatigue and weakness with lightheadedness. They may have symptoms of orthostatic hypotension. Weight loss and nausea and vomiting can occur. The skin may become hyperpigmented with a tan or bronzed appearance. The oral mucosa may have bluish-black patches present. Secretion of the adrenal androgens will also be decreased, sometimes causing a decrease in libido.

Addison's disease should be treated with cortisol replacement therapy. Patients may also require androgen replacement therapy. With secondary adrenal insufficiency, the cause should be the focus of treatment. This could entail resection of a pituitary adenoma. Patients going off steroid therapy should be slowly weaned off the medication to prevent adrenal insufficiency.

Acromegaly

Acromegaly occurs in adults who suffer from excessive production of human growth hormone, usually due to a pituitary adenoma. It can also occur in athletes who treat themselves with high doses of the hormone.

In children, human growth hormone helps with bone growth and development. In adulthood, the epiphyseal plates are closed and the bones are no longer able to grow. With excess human growth hormone, more calcium is laid down on the bone, causing enlargement of the bones. This results in prominent forehead and jawbones, large hands and feet, and arthritis in the spine. Patients may develop left ventricular hypertrophy, CHF, hypertension, and cardiac arrhythmias.

Treatment of acromegaly is aimed at treating the cause. Removal of a pituitary adenoma will decrease or stop the production of human growth hormone. Athletes who use human growth hormone should be urged to discontinue use because of the potential health risks.

Hypopituitary dwarfism

Hypopituitary dwarfism occurs in children who suffer from decreased production of growth hormone. Growth hormone secretion can be decreased in adults, resulting in increased fat and decreased muscle mass, but this will not affect bone growth.

Children who have decreased secretion of human growth hormone, or dwarfism, will be very short in stature because of inadequate bone development. Dwarfism is categorized as a person less than 4'10" tall. These patients are more susceptible to developing sleep apnea and obesity. They may also develop arthritis, decreased flexibility of the joints, scoliosis of the spine, and bowed legs. There are no intellectual deficits associated with dwarfism.

If dwarfism is due to decreased human growth hormone, and not due to a primary skeletal disorder, the child can be treated with human growth hormone treatments to try and stimulate normal growth. Surgery may be necessary to remove a pituitary adenoma if that is the cause of the dwarfism.

Diabetes insipidus

Diabetes insipidus (DI) can have many causes. DI can occur because of increased levels of ADH, or vasopressin, damage to the hypothalamus gland where ADH is produced, damage to the pituitary gland where ADH is stored, or primary kidney damage that prevents the kidneys from functioning properly.

The primary symptoms of diabetes insipidus are increased urinary output with poorly concentrated urine, along with extreme thirst. The increased thirst is due to the increased loss of fluid through the urine and the body's stimulus to replenish this fluid.

The focus of treatment with diabetes insipidus is to treat the underlying cause. Vasopressin can be given nasally or orally to replace the hormone. Hypothalamic tumors can be surgically removed or debulked, if possible. With primary kidney disease, medications should be given to decrease urinary output and prevention dehydration. High-dose anti-inflammatory drugs and diuretics, such as HCTZ, may be helpful.

Type 1 diabetes mellitus

Type 1, insulin-dependent, diabetes mellitus is autoimmune in nature with effects in the islet cells in the pancreas, which cause decreased insulin production. Diabetes mellitus is usually diagnosed early in life, before age 30, and symptoms may come on fairly suddenly. There is <20% chance of family history with this form of diabetes, but a concordance rate in twins.

Patients with type 1 diabetes mellitus will, classically, have symptoms of polyuria and polydipsia. Children may develop bedwetting. There will be weight loss even though patients are eating more, and patients will complain of weakness and fatigue. Diagnosis may be made when patients presents with ketoacidosis or some of the retinal, neurologic, or vascular conditions that accompany diabetes.

Diagnosis is made when fasting blood glucose levels are >126 on two separate occasions, when a 2-hour GTT is >200 on two separate occasions, or when random blood glucose levels are >200 on two separate occasions and symptoms of diabetes are present.

Insulin

The different types of insulin available for controlling glucose levels with type 1 diabetes mellitus are as follows:

Types of Insulin	Onset of Action	Peak Action	Duration of Action
Rapid-acting (Lispro®/Aspart®)	5-15 minutes	1-2 hours	4-6 hours
Short-acting (Regular insulin)	30-60 minutes	2-4 hours	4-10 hours
Intermediate-acting (NPH insulin)	1-2 hours	4-8 hours	10-20 hours
Long-acting (Glargine®)	1-2 hours	No peak	Approx. 24 hours

Type 2 diabetes mellitus

Type 2 diabetes mellitus has its onset later in life, usually after age 30. Its onset is slow and patients often do not know they are diabetic. There is a strong familial tie with this form of diabetes and an even higher twin concordance rate.

Symptoms of this form of diabetes may include polyuria and polydipsia, as with type 1, but these symptoms are not as common. Patients with type 2 diabetes are usually obese. Often times, patients become diagnosed with type 2 diabetes after developing some of the conditions that accompany this condition, such as peripheral vascular disease, peripheral neuropathy, and retinopathy. They may even be in a nonketotic hyperosmolar state at the time of diagnosis.

Treatment of type 2 diabetes is with oral antilipemic agents. There are multiple medications available that can help to suppress glucose formation by the liver or increase the body's sensitivity to insulin. In advanced stages, patients may require insulin therapy to control blood glucose levels.

Controlling glucose levels

There are a number of medications to control glucose levels for type 2 diabetes mellitus:

- Insulin secretagogues – This class of drugs is best utilized in patients who were diagnosed within the last few years. They can decrease the Hgb A1C level by 1-2 points. They should be avoided in renal failure. Side effects include weight gain and hypoglycemia.
- Metformin – This medication is best used in obese patients with insulin resistance. It can decrease the Hgb A1C by 1-2 points. It should be avoided in liver or renal disease, in those with CHF, and before receiving IV contrast. Side effects include nausea, vomiting, diarrhea, and lactic acidosis.
- Glitazones – This class of drugs is best used in obese patients with insulin resistance. It can decrease the Hgb A1C by 0.5-1.5 points. It should be avoided in liver disease and CHF. Side effects include edema, weight gain, anemia, and hepatotoxicity.
- A-glucosidase inhibitors – This class of drugs is best given after meals when glucose levels are highest. It can decrease the Hgb A1C by 0.5-1 points. It should be avoided in intestinal or liver disease. Side effects include flatulence.

Cholesterol

Listed below are the different types of cholesterol and the current recommended guidelines for lipid control:

- Chylomicrons are the least dense particles and are rich in triglycerides.
- Very low-density lipoproteins (VLDL) are made in the liver and are rich in triglycerides.
- Low density lipoproteins (LDL) are rich in cholesterol and are the most arthrogenic.
- High-density lipoproteins (HDL) are rich in cholesterol and are the smallest.
- Treatment goals for hyperlipidemia are based upon CAD risk. They are as follows:
- Low risk (0-1 risk factors): LDL goal is <160. Lifestyle changes should begin with LDL ≥160. Medications should be started with LDL ≥190.
- Moderate risk (2+ risk factors with 10-year risk <10%): LDL goal is <130. Lifestyle changes should begin with LDL ≥130. Medications should be started with LDL ≥160.
- Moderately high risk (2+ risk factors with 10-year risk 10-20%): LDL goal is <130. Lifestyle changes should begin with LDL ≥130. Medication should be started with LDL ≥130.

- High risk (10-year risk >20%): LDL goal is <100. Lifestyle changes should begin with LDL ≥100. Medications should be started with LDL ≥100.

Controlling cholesterol levels

There are a number of medical treatments available to control cholesterol levels:

- Niacin can decrease LDL by 15-25%, can increase HDL by 25-35%, and is very effective at decreasing triglycerides. Side effects include flushing, itching, gout, and peptic ulcers.
- Bile acid-binding resins can decrease LDL by 15-25%, can increase HDL by 5%, and may or may not be helpful with decreasing triglycerides. Side effects include constipation, gas, and decreased fat-soluble vitamin and drug absorption.
- Statins can decrease LDL by 25-50%, increase HDL by 5-15%, and may be quite helpful at decreasing triglycerides. Side effects include myalgias, myositis, and increased liver enzymes.
- Fibrates can decrease LDL by 10-15%, can increase HDL by 15-20%, and are very effective at decreasing triglycerides. Side effects include myalgias, myositis, hepatitis, and gall stones.
- Ezetimibe can decrease LDL by 20%, can increase HDL by 5%, and may or may not be helpful with decreasing triglycerides. Side effects include increased liver enzymes when used in conjunction with a statin.

Gastrointestinal / Nutritional

Esophagitis

When the lower esophageal sphincter becomes lax and does not remain closed properly, the stomach acids can reflux into the esophagus. This causes inflammation in the esophagus, known as esophagitis, eventually leading to ulceration of the mucous membranes lining the esophagus.

Patients will complain of GERD-type symptoms with a burning or bad taste in the throat, pain over the chest into the throat, and possibly a mild cough. They may experience nausea and vomiting. If esophageal ulceration occurs, patients will have severe pain over the chest, worsening with eating. If the ulcer is bleeding, vomiting of blood may occur or the stools may become very dark and tarry. If severe, patients may become anemic due to blood loss.

Treatment of esophagitis often involves lifestyle modifications. These include diet changes to avoid spicy foods, fried foods, and caffeine. Alcohol should be avoided. If patients smoke, they should quit. An H_2-blocker or proton pump inhibitor is given to decrease the acid production in the stomach.

Mallory-Weiss tear

A Mallory-Weiss tear is a laceration of the esophageal mucosa that occurs in the distal portion of the esophagus, near where the esophagus meets the stomach. The tear can be caused by forceful, long-term vomiting or coughing.

Patients will describe an episode of forceful vomiting or coughing followed by vomiting of bright red blood. If this has been going on for a period of time, they may have experienced bloody stools. A past history of a Mallory-Weiss tear may cause a patient to have recurrent incidents of this condition.

Most tears do not need to be surgically corrected. An esophagogastroduodenoscopy (EGD) will be done to confirm diagnosis, and cauterization may be performed if the bleeding has gone on for more than a few hours. Antacids can be given to prevent further irritation of the tear. If there has been significant blood loss, a transfusion may be necessary to correct a volume-depletion anemia.

Esophageal stricture

Damage to the lower esophageal sphincter, either from gastric reflux or some cancers, can cause scarring of the tissue. This scarring can cause the sphincter to be narrowed, which prevents food and fluids from passing into the stomach appropriately.

Patients will complain of difficulty swallowing and a sensation that food is "stuck" in their throat. They may have chest pain and a full feeling. Vomiting can occur if food will not pass into the stomach, especially larger pieces of food.

Treatment of an esophageal stricture involves dilating the sphincter to widen it. This can be accomplished during an EGD by passing dilators, which gradually increase in diameter, through the sphincter. A balloon procedure can also be performed during EGD to widen the sphincter. A risk with both of these procedures is tearing of the esophagus, requiring surgical repair. If these treatments fail to relieve the symptoms, surgery may be needed to correct the sphincter.

Esophageal varices

Esophageal varices almost always occur along with cirrhosis of the liver, but any form of liver disease can lead to their development. With liver disease, blood flow through the organ is obstructed and slowed. This causes portal hypertension, which leads to pressure building in the vessels leading to the organ, and can affect vessels in the esophagus, causing swelling and the formation of varicose veins surrounding the esophagus.

Patients are usually asymptomatic from the esophageal varices themselves but will show signs of liver disease. They may have a history of alcoholism, though not all forms of cirrhosis are caused by alcohol. Other known liver disease may also be present.

Antihypertensives may be given to prevent rupture of the varices, a usually-fatal situation. Anticoagulant medications can be injected into the varices and rubber bands can also be placed around them to prevent rupture. Once rupture occurs, emergency surgery can be performed to try and cauterize the bleeding, but this is usually a futile effort.

GERD

Gastroesophageal reflux disease (GERD) has several different potential causes:

1. Occasional GERD symptoms can be due to consumption of spicy foods or coffee, increased alcohol consumption.
2. Viral gastritis may lead to GERD.
3. Smoking can increase acid production in the stomach and cause GERD.
4. A stressful lifestyle can increase acid production in the stomach.
5. A relaxed lower esophageal sphincter also contributes to GERD symptoms.

Treatment of GERD includes lifestyle modifications with dietary changes, quitting smoking and drinking alcohol, and decreasing daily stress. Avoiding lying down after meals can help. Antacids, H_2-blockers or proton pump inhibitors may be necessary to control the symptoms. Treating GERD symptoms is important to prevent permanent damage to the esophageal mucosa.

Gastric cancer

Gastric cancer can be caused by infection with the *H. pylori* bacteria. This infection causes chronic inflammation in the gastric mucosa, leading to development of cancerous cells in the stomach lining. Eating a diet high in smoked and pickled foods that are high in nitrates may also cause changes in the gastric lining, leading to cancer. Smoking and alcohol use may also play a role in the development of gastric cancer.

Most patients are not aware they have stomach cancer until the disease has progressed to an advanced stage. Most symptoms are similar to GERD-type symptoms and treated at home with antacids. Other symptoms include abdominal pain not relieved by antacids, unintentional weight loss, chronic feeling of fullness, and tarry stools if bleeding is occurring. Patients may develop a blockage within the stomach with a large tumor that prevents them from eating.

Treatment is with surgical removal of the malignant tissue. Radiation and chemotherapy may be necessary.

Peptic ulcer disease

Peptic ulcer disease occurs in the stomach or duodenum and has several causes. Infection with *H. pylori* bacteria can lead to ulcers. Excessive acid production in the stomach due to a tumor can also break down the gastric mucosa and cause ulcers. The most common cause of peptic ulcer disease is the use of anti-inflammatory medications, like ibuprofen and naproxen. Aspirin use can be caustic to the stomach and cause ulcers.

Patients will complain of abdominal pain. The pain may be relieved with eating as food coats the stomach, though spicy foods can aggravate the pain. Patients may feel bloated and have nausea and vomiting. With bleeding of the ulcer, stools may be tarry, and there may be blood in vomitus. Treatment is focused on treating the cause. NSAIDs should be stopped if this is the cause. Infection with *H. pylori* should be treated with a combination of antibiotics and an antacid. Dietary changes to reduce acid secretion are recommended. Surgery is necessary if the ulcer has perforated.

Pyloric stenosis

Pyloric stenosis occurs in infants when the pylorus, or opening between the stomach and duodenum, becomes enlarged. This prevents the transport of food from the stomach to the small intestine. Though there is no definite known cause, it is thought it may be genetic in nature. It is also thought that this condition develops after birth and not *in utero*.

The infant will have gradually worsening vomiting after meals. Projectile vomiting is not uncommon, and the child will act fussy and hungry even after eating. Constipation is common, and dehydration will eventually develop. The infant will also show a slower degree of weight gain and may begin losing weight. On exam, an olive-shaped mass can be palpated in the abdomen due to the enlarged pylorus.

Treatment is by surgical correction of the pyloric sphincter. This is usually a very successful surgery that results in full recovery from the condition.

Cholecystitis

Cholecystitis is an inflammatory condition of the gallbladder, occurring because bile builds up in the organ, leading to inflammation, swelling, and infection. The bile normally passes from the gallbladder to the small intestine to aid in digestion, but there is a disruption in this flow with cholecystitis. Usually this disruption is due to gallstones.

Cholecystitis is more likely to occur in females than males, and patients are frequently overweight. Patients will develop severe abdominal pain that is often present after eating a fatty meal. This pain is often aggravated with taking a deep breath. There may be bloating, nausea, and vomiting present. Oftentimes patients will complain of referred right shoulder pain. Abdominal ultrasound will often reveal gallstones, though a CT scan may be necessary.

Treatment is with a cholecystectomy, usually done laparoscopically when possible. Some patients may have occasional flare-ups of cholecystitis that resolve spontaneously.

Cholelithiasis

Cholelithiasis is the development of gallstones from cholesterol and other fatty byproducts within the gallbladder. These can block the ducts leading from the gallbladder, causing cholecystitis.

Symptoms can vary depending on which duct is blocked by the stone. Ducts leading to the pancreas can cause acute pancreatitis with severe abdominal pain and vomiting. Blockage of ducts leading to the liver can result in jaundice. Generally, patients will experience nausea and vomiting, abdominal pain that may refer to the right shoulder, and bloating.

Patients may have several flare-ups of pain from the gallstones and may hold off on having surgery. Some patients can have gallstones and be asymptomatic. Patients who do not undergo surgery for correction of this condition should be advised to avoid fatty foods that can aggravate the problem and contribute to enlargement of the gallstones or development of new stones. Cholecystectomy to remove the gallbladder and stones and removal of a stone from a duct may be necessary.

Hepatitis

Hepatitis can be divided into three categories:

- Hepatitis A is a viral infection of the liver that is transmitted through the fecal-oral route by infected individuals and can be contracted through contaminated food and water, especially raw shellfish. It causes abdominal pain, nausea and vomiting, and jaundice. Arthritis may also develop. Symptoms generally resolve spontaneously within 2 months.
- Hepatitis B is a blood-borne viral infection and is contracted through contact with blood and body fluids of infected individuals. It causes abdominal pain, nausea and vomiting, jaundice, and may lead to liver failure. Treatment is usually limited to symptomatic control and the condition usually resolves on its own. Chronic conditions are treated with interferon or lamivudine.
- Hepatitis C is also contracted through blood and body fluids. It is the most serious form of viral hepatitis and is the leading cause of liver transplants. The symptoms are the same as the other

forms of viral hepatitis, though liver failure or liver cancer can develop. Treatment is generally with pegylated interferon and ribavirin.

Cirrhosis

Cirrhosis of the liver is most often caused by alcoholism. Chronic viral hepatitis and some autoimmune conditions can also cause cirrhosis. Scarring forms in the liver, decreasing the ability of the liver to function properly. As cirrhosis progresses, liver function decreases, and patients eventually develop liver failure. There is a high mortality rate with cirrhosis.

Patients will develop an enlarged liver early on due to inflammation, but then the liver will shrink as scar tissue develops. Patients will develop ascites and portal hypertension. Esophageal varices can develop. Electrolyte abnormalities, along with clotting disorders, can also develop.

Treatment of cirrhosis should focus on treating the cause. Alcoholics should obtain proper treatment to help them stop drinking. The symptoms should be treated by correcting electrolyte imbalances and coagulating esophageal varices. A liver transplant may eventually be necessary, but only in patients who have abstained from alcohol for a significant amount of time.

Pancreatitis

The most common cause of pancreatitis is excessive alcohol consumption, in both binge drinkers and chronic alcoholics. Pancreatitis can also occur from cholelithiasis and associated duct blockage. Some autoimmune disorders, such as cystic fibrosis, can also leave patients susceptible to pancreatitis. High triglyceride levels can cause a patient to be more susceptible to developing pancreatitis.

Symptoms include severe abdominal pain that radiates into the back. Patients may have intractable vomiting. Electrolyte imbalances can develop due to the lack of digestive enzymes in the stomach.

Treatment of pancreatitis is mostly symptomatic. Patients should be NPO, and tube feedings though a nasogastric tube may be necessary. This allows the pancreas to rest and heal. IV fluids and correction of electrolyte imbalances are necessary. Sometimes the damage to the pancreas is severe enough to warrant surgical resection of a portion of the organ. Patients may go on to develop a chronic form of the disease.

Appendicitis

Appendicitis occurs due to blockage and inflammation of the appendix from feces or a foreign body. Certain forms of cancer can also cause inflammation of the organ. Blockage of the appendix will lead to swelling, inflammation, infection, and abscess formation. Appendicitis should be surgically treated immediately to prevent eventual rupture of the organ and subsequent peritonitis.

Patients will complain of periumbilical pain that gradually worsens and eventually migrates to the right lower abdomen. Nausea and vomiting are usually present early on. Fever may also be present. A CT scan or ultrasound may show an enlarged appendix. The WBC will be elevated, possibly up to 15,000.

If the diagnosis is not confirmed with CT or ultrasound, but other possible diseases that could cause patients' symptoms have been ruled out, the organ is still usually removed to prevent the potential rupture of the appendix. The appendectomy can usually be performed laparoscopically.

Diverticulitis

Diverticula are outpouchings in the large intestine that commonly develop during the aging process. This is due to weakening of the intestinal walls with decreased smooth muscle integrity. Diverticulitis occurs when digestive matter becomes trapped within these outpouchings, leading to swelling, inflammation, and infection. Diverticula can rupture if the condition becomes severe.

Patients will generally complain of left lower abdominal pain. Patients may complain of bloating and gas with diarrhea. Nausea and vomiting may be present, along with fever.
Diverticulitis is generally treated with IV fluids and antibiotics. Patients should be kept NPO and receive feedings through a nasogastric tube. Diverticulitis usually resolves without surgery, but resection of the affected portion of the intestine may be necessary in severe cases.

Intussusception

Intussusception is a telescoping of the small intestine or colon that causes blood flow to be blocked and prevents the movement of food and feces through the bowel. It usually occurs in children, rarely in adults, and there is usually no known cause.

Children will have nausea, vomiting, and fever. They may have diarrhea with "currant jelly" stools because of the frank blood that is present. There will be abdominal pain that may be severe, but it can be intermittent. On exam, there may be a palpable mass in the abdomen and abdominal tenderness.

Treatment of intussusception is usually successful with a barium or air enema. This forces the bowel to straighten and slides the telescoped portion of the bowel back to normal. If there is damaged or dead tissue, surgery may be necessary to resect the ischemic portion of bowel. Most children recover well after treatment without recurrence of the condition.

Irritable bowel syndrome

Irritable bowel syndrome (IBS) is very common and may affect up to 20% of Americans. It usually occurs in response to stressors, either psychological or physical, and can be severe enough to be debilitating.

Patients will complain of intermittent periods of bloating, painful gas, and alternating diarrhea and constipation. Some patients may have predominantly diarrhea or constipation while others alternate between the two. A pattern of symptoms may be discernible after people eat certain foods or during periods of stress. Chronic illness may also cause IBS and lead to flare-ups of the condition.

Fiber supplements to bulk the stool can help with the constipation while antidiarrheals may help with the diarrhea. Avoiding the triggering factors that lead to flare-ups can also help control symptoms. If chronic illness is the cause, managing the illness to prevent episodes of IBS can be helpful. There is research being conducted on medications specifically formulated to treat the symptoms of IBS.

Ulcerative colitis

Ulcerative colitis is an inflammatory disease that affects the mucous membranes lining the rectum and large intestine. The cause of ulcerative colitis is not clearly understood, but it is thought that to be immune-mediated due to infection with a virus or bacteria. There is a genetic-tendency for the disease, also. Ulcerative colitis is not caused by stress though this can aggravate the symptoms of ulcerative colitis. Patients will complain of abdominal pain with diarrhea. There may be obvious blood in the stool. Many people experience a spasm of the rectum, causing an urge to defecate but inability to do so.

Treatment is with anti-inflammatory drugs and sometimes short-term steroids to help control the inflammation within the colon. There are immunosuppressant medications available that will help suppress flare-ups of the condition. Antidiarrheals and pain relievers may also be helpful. If mucosal damage is severe, surgery may be necessary to resect the damaged portion of the large intestine.

Crohn's disease

Crohn's disease is an inflammatory condition that can affect any portion of the digestive tract, from the mouth to the anus. It causes breaks in the mucosal lining of the tract, and patients may experience periods of remission during which the symptoms are not present. The cause of Crohn's disease is not known, but it is thought to be due to a bacterial infection, an autoimmune response, or possibly genetic factors.

Patients with Crohn's disease will complain of abdominal pain with or without fever and poor appetite. There may be evident weight loss with the disease. Patients frequently have diarrhea, possibly with blood present. Because Crohn's disease can occur at any point in the digestive tract, symptoms may be more focused on a particular area, such as the mouth or anus.

There is no cure for Crohn's disease. Treatment is symptomatic with the goal being to reduce inflammation within the digestive tract. This can be accomplished with anti-inflammatory drugs, possibly steroids, and antibiotics.

Bowel obstruction

A bowel obstruction can be caused by improper function of the organ or by mechanical obstruction. An ileus is not caused by mechanical obstruction. It can be due to medications, infection, ischemia, injury, or manipulation during surgery. Mechanical obstruction of the bowel can occur from tumors, adhesions, hernias, or impacted stool.

Patients will complain of abdominal pain and cramping in the absence of regular bowel movements or gas. They may have vomiting and a full, bloated feeling. On exam, bowel sounds may be high-pitched or tingling in nature early on, but eventually there will be absent bowel sounds.

Treatment of a bowel obstruction involves resting the bowel. A nasogastric tube will be inserted and set to low suction to decompress the gut. This often improves patients' sensations of bloating and stops the vomiting. If the condition is severe, a portion of bowel may need to be resected, especially if blood flow is compromised or if a severe infection develops.

Toxic megacolon

Toxic megacolon usually occurs in those patients who suffer from inflammatory bowel disease. It results in a distended colon and can be a life-threatening condition.

Patients may complain of abdominal distention and pain, with or without fever. Toxic megacolon can progress to the development of shock symptoms. Patients may appear dehydrated and have a rapid heart rate. Abdominal x-rays will show the dilated colon. WBC may be elevated and potassium may be decreased if patients are dehydrated.

The colon is rested for 24 hours to try and reduce the distention. If this is not affective, surgery is usually done to resect that section of the colon. This condition can lead to shock and death, so prompt treatment is necessary. Patients should be hydrated with IV fluids and any electrolyte imbalances should be corrected. Steroids may be given to reduce inflammation within the organ and antibiotics will be useful if patients become septic.

Anal fissure

An anal fissure is a small tear in the tissue surrounding the anal sphincter. It is caused by excessive stretching of the anal sphincter, as with a large bowel movement.

Patients will complain of pain at the anus, especially with bowel movements. They may have noticed bright red blood in their stool or on toilet paper following a bowel movement. There may also be a history of constipation present. A rectal exam will be extremely painful for these patients. The anal sphincter should be visually assessed to identify the anal fissure.

Anal fissures usually resolve without treatment. If the fissures are very painful, Sitz baths may be soothing. A topical anesthetic can be used if the pain is preventing patients from having a bowel movement. To prevent recurrence, stool softeners and a diet high in fiber and fluids should be recommended to keep bowel movements regular and prevent constipation.

Anorectal abscess

An anorectal abscess, or infection in the anal or rectal areas, can have several causes. An anal fissure can become infected, or an anal gland can become blocked, leading to abscess formation. Anal sexual intercourse can also place a patient at risk for developing an anorectal abscess.

An anorectal abscess will cause patients significant pain with the development of an indurated, inflamed area near the anus. This may feel like a hard, hot lump at the edge of the anus. Patients may have very painful bowel movements or may develop constipation because of the fear of having a bowel movement. If the abscess ruptures, pus may be discharged through the rectum.

The abscess will need to be drained and if it is deep or very extensive, surgery may be necessary. Sitz baths can help with some of the inflammation, and antibiotics will be necessary to help cure the infection.

Hemorrhoids

Hemorrhoids occur when the veins surrounding the anus and rectum become engorged and swollen. Hemorrhoids commonly occur with excessive straining with a bowel movement, such as when constipated, and during pregnancy because of the increased pressure applied to the pelvic floor. Hemorrhoids can also occur as a result of anal sexual intercourse and as part of the aging process. Hemorrhoids can be internal or external.

Internal hemorrhoids can bleed and will cause patients to have bright red blood on the toilet paper after a bowel movement. If hemorrhoids protrude through the anus, they will be painful. External hemorrhoids are visibly noticeable and occur on the outside of the anus. They are painful and may itch or bleed.

Most hemorrhoids will resolve without treatment, but topical ointments are available to help relieve the swelling and pain. Sitz baths can also help to relieve the inflammation. If severe or recurrent, surgery may be necessary to remove the hemorrhoids.

Pilonidal cyst

A pilonidal cyst is a cyst that forms at the base of the coccyx and becomes infected. It occurs at the superior end of the cleft between the buttocks. Pilonidal cysts occur in equal numbers of men and women.

Some believe that a pilonidal cyst occurs due to ingrown hair in the region. Another theory is that it may be due to repeated trauma in the sacral and coccyx area. The cyst will form like a typical abscess with a red, indurated area at the base of the spine. Patients may or may not have a fever, but the cyst will be painful. If it opens, pus will drain from the cyst.

As initial treatment, warm Sitz baths may help to prevent abscess formation. If an abscess does continue to develop, antibiotics may be given to resolve the infection. If this is not effective, surgical incision and drainage will be necessary, followed by oral antibiotics.

Hernias

There are different types of hernias:

- Hiatal hernias occur when the upper segment of the stomach protrudes through the diaphragm, causing a telescoping affect around the distal esophagus.
- Incisional hernias occur at the site of an abdominal surgical incision and result in a portion of bowel protruding through the abdominal wall.
- Inguinal hernias occur in the groin through a weakened portion of the inguinal canal.
- Umbilical hernias occur at the umbilicus due to a weakened area of the abdominal fascia, causing the bowel to protrude through the umbilical opening.
- Ventral hernias can occur anywhere there is a weakened area in the abdominal wall; they cause a section of bowel to protrude through the opening.
- Hernias are treated surgically. Hiatal hernias may require a Nissan fundoplication procedure in which the lower esophagus is reinforced with mesh to strengthen the area surrounding it, preventing the stomach from extending up around the esophagus. All other hernias are repaired by weaving a mesh material at the site of the weakened area to strengthen the wall.

Vitamin deficiencies

<u>Niacin</u>

A niacin, or vitamin B_3, deficiency can lead to a condition called pellagra. This can occur due to malnutrition with a lack of niacin in the diet, or because of a malabsorption syndrome that prevents the body from absorbing niacin. The "3 D's" can occur with advanced pellagra:

1. Dementia.
2. Diarrhea.
3. Dermatitis.

Patients may experience weakness and have obvious signs of malnutrition, such as weight loss. Excoriations and signs of inflammation can be present on the skin. Patients may be irritable or short-tempered before the dementia becomes evident.

Treatment of a niacin deficiency involves replacing the niacin so patients have normal serum levels of the vitamin. If malabsorption is the cause of the deficiency, measures should be taken to correct this condition if possible. Carcinoid or other gastric tumors may cause obstruction that prevents absorption of the niacin, and these should be surgically removed, if possible, to allow absorption.

Vitamin A

Vitamin A is a fat-soluble vitamin and is helpful in boosting the immune system as well as help with maintaining bone and teeth integrity. Vitamin A helps to keep the eyes healthy and makes night vision possible. It is thought that vitamin A may help to prevent some forms of cancer.

A primary vitamin A deficiency can be due to malnutrition and is rare in developed countries. Malabsorption systems that prevent absorption of fats may prevent absorption of vitamin A. Deficiency in vitamin A can lead to diarrhea, infection, respiratory disorders, night blindness and eventual complete blindness. Skin disorders can also occur with a lack of vitamin A.

Vitamin A deficiency is treated by giving supplemental vitamin A. If a malabsorption syndrome is the cause of the deficiency, this should be corrected if possible. Disorders that disrupt the absorption of fat, necessary for vitamin A absorption, should be treated if possible.

Riboflavin

Riboflavin, or vitamin B_2, is a water-soluble vitamin. It is necessary for normal cell growth, development, and energy production. Riboflavin also helps in red blood cell production.

A deficiency in riboflavin may be due to malnutrition, though this is rare in industrialized countries. It can also be caused by a malabsorption syndrome that prevents riboflavin from being absorbed.

Symptoms of riboflavin deficiency include swelling of the mucous membranes, sore throat, and canker sores on the lips or in the mouth. Dermatitis may develop without adequate levels of riboflavin, as can certain types of anemia. If due to malnutrition, obvious muscle wasting and weight loss will be evident.

Treatment is by replacement with riboflavin. If there is an underlying malabsorption disorder causing the deficiency, then this should be treated if possible. Riboflavin is excreted from the body through urine. There are no known cases of poisoning by riboflavin from taking excess supplements or by consuming too many foods high in riboflavin.

Vitamin C

Vitamin C is a vital substance that all humans need to prevent illness. It is responsible for the proper formation of blood vessels and is useful in wound healing. It is also necessary for cartilage formation. A deficiency in vitamin C causes an illness known as scurvy. Historically, this was seen in those who were at sea for extended periods of time and did not have access to foods rich in vitamin C. Scurvy causes discoloration of the skin, similar to liver spots. It also causes breakdown of collagen and some connective tissues, leading to tooth loss and immobility. The skin can easily break down and form ulcerative wounds if a person does not have adequate vitamin C intake, and this can eventually lead to death.

Treatment of a vitamin C deficiency requires dietary changes that increase a person's consumption of foods rich in vitamin C, such as citrus fruit. Supplements are also available to help with replacement of the vitamin.

Vitamin D

Vitamin D is a fat-soluble vitamin that plays a vital role in calcium absorption into the bones to provide healthy, strong teeth and bones. Vitamin D is readily found in dairy products and fish.

A deficiency of vitamin D leads to a condition called rickets in children and osteoporosis in adults. Rickets will produce a bowing of the legs of children because of bone softening. Bone growth will also be stifled without vitamin D. Osteoporosis in adults places these individuals at higher risk of developing a compression fracture or large bone fracture because of brittle bones.

Vitamin D supplements are available, often combined with calcium, for those who require extra doses of the vitamin. Increasing dairy products and fortified foods in the diet will also increase vitamin D intake. Vitamin D is known as the "sunshine vitamin" and is produced within the skin after exposure to sunlight. Daily sun exposure (15-20 minutes) can help increase a person's vitamin D level.

Vitamin K

Vitamin K is a fat-soluble vitamin that is found in abundant supply in green, leafy vegetables. It plays a vital role in the clotting cascade to prevent excessive bleeding. A deficiency in vitamin K is very rare, but it can be seen in those individuals with a form of malabsorption syndrome that prevents that absorption of fats from the GI tract. This will lead to a decrease in the amount of vitamin K that is absorbed from foods. The blood thinning drug warfarin (Coumadin®) blocks the function of vitamin K in the clotting cascade, which promotes bleeding and a decreased clotting time.

Treatment of a vitamin K deficiency can be reversed with injectable vitamin K. This is also given to infants shortly after birth to help prevent excessive bleeding. A malabsorption syndrome that prevents absorption of fats from the digestive tract should be treated, if possible, to prevent the malabsorption of vitamin K.

Lactose intolerance

Lactose intolerance develops in those individuals who are lacking in the enzyme lactase, which breaks down the sugar in milk. There are no known specific causes for lactose intolerance.

Patients will complain of bloating or abdominal pain shortly after eating dairy foods. There can also be cramping diarrhea, which is very common, along with nausea. Patients may have painful gas.

Diagnosis of true lactose intolerance can be done in a few different ways. Patients can be tested after fasting overnight and given a dairy-rich drink. The blood is then measured over two hours to assess glucose levels. If the glucose levels remain low, there is a deficiency in lactase. Another test is by giving a lactose-rich drink to patients and the measure hydrogen levels in the breath. These should remain low, but will be elevated with lactose intolerance.

Treatment is with dietary changes to avoid lactose-rich foods and beverages. Calcium supplementation may be necessary to ensure patients are receiving adequate amounts.

Phenylketonuria

Phenylketonuria, or PKU, is a disorder in which an infant is not able to digest phenylalanine, a protein found in most foods. This causes phenylalanine to accumulate in the bloodstream and leads to severe brain damage and mental retardation.

Screening is done nationwide at birth to identify infants suffering from this condition. Patients who do have PKU may have lighter skin and hair because phenylalanine helps to produce melanin in the body. These children will be developmentally delayed and show signs of mental retardation. They are more likely to suffer from a seizure disorder, jerky movements, and hyperactivity.

PKU can be treated, but early identification is necessary. All children should be tested at birth for the presence of PKU. If PKU is diagnosed, a diet very low in phenylalanine should be strictly followed. If this is adhered to, mental retardation can be mild and there may be minimal impairment in function. If this diet is not closely followed, mental retardation will result.

Genitourinary

Benign prostatic hyperplasia

Benign prostatic hyperplasia, or BPH, is a benign enlargement of the prostate gland. There is no definite known cause though it may be familial. Whenever there is a change in the size of the prostate gland, a complete assessment should be done to ensure it is not cause by a malignancy.

Patients will complain of urinary frequency or urgency. Oftentimes they may have to urinate frequently, but only in small amounts. There may also be dribbling present at the end of the urinary stream and a decrease in the force of the urinary stream. Patients may have recurrent urinary tract infections. The prostate gland will feel smooth and enlarged on rectal exam, and the PSA is mildly elevated.

Treatment is with medications that help slow the growth of the prostate, such as Flomax® or Hytrin®. If symptoms are severe, surgery may be necessary to remove a portion of the prostate.

Cryptorchidism

Cryptorchidism occurs when one or both of the testicles fail to descend into the scrotum. This can be due to prematurity, low birth weight, or hormone balance abnormalities. In most boys, the testes will descend within the first 3 months of life. Cryptorchidism resolves in most infants by the first birthday, but about 1% of infants will not have resolution.

The symptoms, obviously, are the absence of one or more testes from the scrotum. The initial newborn exam includes palpating the scrotum to feel that both testes are there. They may be palpable a little further up the inguinal canal on one or both sides. Repeated checks should be done at follow-up visits to ensure the testicles descend.

Treatment of cryptorchidism involves surgery to force the testes to descend into the scrotum. Hormonal treatments with HCG may be helpful to naturally cause them to descend. There is an increased risk of infertility and testicular cancer in patients who suffer from true cryptorchidism.

Hydrocele

A hydrocele is a collection of fluid in the scrotum, surrounding the testicles. This is most common in infant boys and usually absorbs within the first year of life. Occasionally, the fluid does not absorb because the fluid is not able to flow back into the abdomen. A hydrocele can also occur in adult males, usually over 40, due to an injury or infection.

Patients do not usually have any pain in the scrotum when a hydrocele is present. Pain will be present if an infection is the cause, or if there has been an injury to the scrotum. The main concern patients will have is of the enlargement of the scrotum.

Most of the time, a hydrocele will resolve spontaneously. Rarely, surgery may be necessary to remove the hydrocele from the scrotum. A fine needle aspiration can also be done to drain the fluid from the scrotum.

Varicocele

A varicocele is an engorgement of the veins of the pampiniform plexus. This plexus is part of the spermatic cord that travels through the inguinal canal, terminating in the testes. A varicocele is more likely to occur in the left testis because the veins from there run vertically into the renal vein. The veins from the right testis empty into the inferior vena cava.

A varicocele is usually idiopathic in nature but can be caused by compression preventing the veins from draining. This condition usually occurs in males ages 15-25, but a malignant tumor should be considered in patients who develop a varicocele after the age of 40.

Patients will complain of a heavy, aching, fullness in the affected testicle. On exam, the testicle may appear visibly enlarged with engorged veins. When palpated, the testicle may feel like a "bag of worms."

A scrotal support may be used to try and resolve the condition on its own. If this is not effective, surgery may be necessary.

Paraphimosis

Paraphimosis is a condition that occurs in the uncircumcised male. It occurs when the foreskin of the penis becomes trapped behind the glans. The foreskin can normally be retracted manually and will slide back over the glans on its own or with little effort. The foreskin will become edematous and patients will complain of pain from the constriction. Paraphimosis can cause compromise of the blood flow and may lead to gangrene if untreated.

A lubricant can be used to assist in sliding the foreskin over the glans to its normal position. The Dundee technique, in which a small gauge needle is used to create punctures in the foreskin, can also be used. The edematous fluid is then compressed from the tissue so the foreskin can be slid down. If these procedures fail, surgery may be necessary to create a slit in the foreskin to enable it to slide back to its normal position. A circumcision should be performed in these patients to prevent reoccurrence.

Testicular torsion

The testicle is usually held in place by the tunica vaginalis, which allows little movement. Some males are born with a congenital anomaly that allows the testicles to move easily and rotate horizontally on the spermatic cord. This leaves them susceptible to developing testicular torsion in which a testicle can twist on the spermatic cord. This causes obstruction of blood flow to the testicle.

Patients will complain of a sudden, severe testicular pain. This may occur after activity or while sleeping. Trauma may also contribute to a testicular torsion. The testicle may appear swollen or discolored, and the affected testicle may appear elevated when compared to the other. Patients may have nausea and vomiting.

Treatment should be emergent because of the risk of tissue death from decreased blood flow. The torsion may be resolved by manually manipulating the testicle back into a normal position, but surgery may be necessary. With tissue death, an orchiectomy may be performed.

Cystitis

Cystitis, or a urinary tract infection (UTI), is an infection of the bladder. It is more common in women because of an anatomically shorter urethra, but can also occur in men. It is most common in women aged 30-50 and in men over 50 because of enlargement of the prostate obstructing urine flow. A UTI is caused by bacteria that travel up the urethra to the bladder to multiply. Women are more susceptible to developing a UTI after frequent sexual intercourse because of exposure to bacteria.

Symptoms include burning on urination and frequent urination of small amounts of urine. Patients may have lower abdominal pain with or without a fever. Urinalysis will show WBCs and RBCs, positive nitrates, and bacteria. Culture and sensitivity should be done to isolate the causative organism, which are frequently *Escherichia coli*.

Appropriate antibiotic therapy should be given for treatment. Urethral anesthetizing medications can be given to reduce the pain. Patients should have another urinalysis after treatment is completed to ensure the infection is resolved.

Epididymitis

The epididymis is located on the posterior surface of each testicle and functions to store sperm. It can become inflamed and infected, resulting in epididymitis. Epididymitis is most common in males under age 35 and is frequently due to a bacterial infection from a sexually transmitted disease, such as chlamydia or gonorrhea. Patients will complain of pain in the affected testicle, exacerbated with straining, such as with a bowel movement. They may also have pain with urinating and lower abdominal pain. There may be visible blood in the semen with pain on ejaculation. High fever and chills are common, along with enlarged inguinal lymph nodes. The testicle will feel warm and swollen with a palpable enlarged epididymis.

Appropriate antibiotics are given to treat the infection. Patients should be counseled on condom use to prevent future STDs. Rarely, an abscess may form that requires drainage or even removal of part of the epididymis.

Prostatitis

Inflammation or infection of the prostate gland may be acute or chronic. Acute prostatitis is usually caused by a bacterial infection. Chronic prostatitis can be due to inflammation from a variety of causes, including urine backing up into the gland causing inflammation, interstitial cystitis, or spasms of the urinary sphincters.

Patients with either form of prostatitis will complain of lower abdominal pain and pain on ejaculation, but a fever will be much more pronounced in patients with the acute form of the condition. Urinary frequency, decreased stream, and urgency will be present with both. On exam, the prostate gland will feel boggy and enlarged. Patients with acute prostatitis will have severe pain with palpation of the gland.

Treatment is with appropriate antibiotics and analgesics. Chronic prostatitis may benefit from muscle relaxants and anti-inflammatory agents. Surgery may be necessary to remove all or a portion of the prostate if the symptoms of chronic prostatitis cannot be controlled.

Pyelonephritis

Pyelonephritis is a severe infection of the kidneys. Pyelonephritis can be life-threatening if not treated promptly. Chronic renal damage, which may impair renal function, can occur without treatment. Commonly, pyelonephritis is caused by a urinary tract infection (UTI) that spreads from the bladder, through the ureters, and to the kidneys.

The symptoms of pyelonephritis are similar to a UTI, only more severe. Urinary frequency, urgency, decreased stream, painful burning on urination, lower abdominal pain, and foul-smelling urine are present. Patients may have a high fever with chills. On exam, there will be pain to percussion over the costovertebral angle over the kidneys. Urinalysis will show elevated WBCs and RBCs with many bacteria.

Treatment is with appropriate antibiotic therapy, usually a broad-spectrum antibiotic such as amoxicillin or a quinolone. If severe, patients may require hospitalization with IV antibiotics. There is a risk of urosepsis with pyelonephritis, so treatment should begin immediately after diagnosis.

Wilms tumor

A Wilms tumor, or nephroblastoma, is a renal carcinoma that affects children usually ages 3-8. It is thought that a Wilms tumor begins to form while *in utero*. Some of the cells that would normally develop into renal cells fail to develop, and this mutation goes on to form a tumor. The condition is usually diagnosed by age 1, though sometimes it may be as late as age 5.

Often a mass can be palpated in the abdomen and in the back over the affected kidney. A Wilms tumor can grow large before causing any pain in the child, so it may go undiagnosed until it becomes large enough to be palpable. There will frequently be visible blood in the urine. The child may become constipated and have nausea and vomiting. This may be accompanied by weight loss.

Treatment comprises surgery, chemotherapy, and radiation, or a combination of all three treatments.

Acute glomerulonephritis

Acute glomerulonephritis is an infection of the kidneys that affects the glomerular filters within the organs. It is usually sudden in onset and can lead to permanent kidney damage of not treated promptly. The cause of acute glomerulonephritis can be *streptococcal* infection, virus, or occur bacterial endocarditis.

Patients will be acutely ill with glomerulonephritis. They will have a decrease in urinary output with a dark tea-stain color to their urine due to hematuria. The urine may appear foamy because of a high protein level. Edema can be quite profound, affecting the extremities and face. Blood pressure will be elevated due to the increased fluid load. Urinalysis will show elevated RBCs, WBCs with infection, and elevated protein levels.

Treatment will focus on treating the underlying cause. If due to a recent *streptococcal* infection or bacterial endocarditis, appropriate antibiotic therapy should be prescribed. The condition will usually resolve on its own with management of the symptoms, such as ACE inhibitors to control hypertension and diuretics to reduce the edema.

Nephrotic syndrome

Nephrotic syndrome is a condition that occurs due to damage to the microvascular system within the kidneys. It leads to excess excretion of protein in the urine and leaking of serum proteins out of the vessels, causing edema. There is also an increased risk of blood clot development. Nephrotic syndrome can be caused by chronic renal failure that occurs due to a primary renal disease or diabetic nephropathy. Other chronic conditions that can cause nephrotic syndrome include lupus erythematosus and amyloidosis.

Nephrotic syndrome can cause a good deal of edema, especially in the extremities and face. There may be noticeable weight gain due to the retained fluid. Patients will have a feeling of general malaise and may or may not have a fever. Urinalysis will show very high levels of protein.

Treatment focuses on treating the underlying cause and controlling the symptoms of nephrotic syndrome. ACE inhibitors can be given to control hypertension and diuretics to reduce the edema. Anticoagulants may be necessary to prevent blood clot formation.

Polycystic kidney disease

Polycystic kidney disease is a condition in which groups of cysts form within the kidneys. It can potentially lead to high blood pressure and even renal failure. Polycystic disease is not limited to the kidneys and can affect other organs as well, but the kidneys are usually the most severely affected. This is a genetic condition that can be autosomal dominant or autosomal recessive.

Patients may complain of abdominal pain and an increasing abdominal girth due to enlarging kidneys. They may have frequent urination or gross blood visible in the urine. High blood pressure is usually present and early signs of renal failure may be evident with elevated serum BUN and creatinine levels.

Treatment of polycystic kidney disease is focused on treating the symptoms and preventing renal failure. Close monitoring and control of blood pressure is necessary. If the cysts become large, they may need to be surgically drained to prevent compression on surrounding organs.

Hyponatremia

Hyponatremia can be due to syndrome of inappropriate antidiuretic hormone secretion (SIADH) and suddenly stopping steroid treatment without tapering the medication. Hypomagnesemia can also cause a decrease in sodium levels. Mild hyponatremia will result in nausea and vomiting and other vague flu-like symptoms. Moderate hyponatremia causes muscular effects of weakness and muscle pain. Severe hyponatremia causes changes in mental status with lethargy and psychosis. If severe, seizures can occur that may lead to coma and possibly even death.

Decreases in the sodium level may be the result of dilutional effects from over-hydration. Fluid restrictions can be implemented to return the sodium levels to normal. If hyponatremia is severe, IV fluids with high sodium content can be administered along with a diuretic to increase fluid output. If an abnormality in the amount of ADH is present, as with SIADH, an antibiotic can be given to correct this. If the SIADH is due to malignancy, treatment of the cancer can help to correct the condition. Significant diuresis may be necessary if fluid overload is causing a dilutional hyponatremia.

Hypernatremia

Hypernatremia can be caused by a decrease in fluid intake or dehydration. Diabetes insipidus can result in changes in antidiuretic hormone levels, which can alter sodium regulation. Renal dysfunction can alter the excretion of sodium and result in higher levels within the blood stream. Hypermagnesemia can also cause an increase in sodium levels.

If renal dysfunction is contributing to increased water wasting, increased urinary output will be present. If dehydration is the cause, excessive sweating and dryness of the oral mucosa can be present. Patients may have had some nausea and vomiting with a decrease in oral fluid intake if that is the cause of the dehydration. Nervous system effects include changes in mental status with irritability, somnolence, or seizures. Deep tendon reflexes may be depressed. Patients should be treated for dehydration if this is the cause and IV fluids provided to correct the imbalance if the renal system will allow this. If caused by increases in magnesium levels, then the hypermagnesemia should be treated.

Hypokalemia

Hypokalemia is defined as a potassium level <3.5. Increased excretion of potassium, such as with diuretics or with dehydration through diarrhea and vomiting, can cause decreased levels of potassium. Various antibiotics can also cause hypokalemia. Because potassium and sodium have an inverse relationship, an increase in sodium levels can cause hypokalemia.

Hypokalemia can cause cardiac dysrhythmias and an increased heart rate. Decreased blood pressure may be present along with mental status changes, such as somnolence or even seizures. If potassium levels drop severely low, fatal cardiac dysrhythmias can occur with cardiac arrest. EKG changes include flattened T waves and ST depression, similar to cardiac ischemia.

Treatment is with IV solutions with added potassium chloride. Potassium-rich foods can be given to increase intake of potassium. Patients must be closely monitored for signs and symptoms of hyperkalemia as potassium supplements are given, especially cardiac effects. Other electrolyte levels, especially sodium, should be closely monitored for abnormalities.

Hyperkalemia

Hyperkalemia is defined as a potassium level >5.5. Potassium is excreted through urine so any dysfunction that results in a decreased urinary output can cause increased serum potassium levels. Any process that causes blood cell destruction, such as hemolytic anemia, can cause a rise in potassium levels. Various medications can also lead to hyperkalemia.

Neuromuscular symptoms of weakness, lethargy, diminished reflexes, and tingling of the extremities may occur. Hyperkalemia causes a decreased heart rate and cardiac dysrhythmias. EKG changes include a wide QRS complex and elevated T waves. GI symptoms of nausea, vomiting, and diarrhea may be present.

Treatment is achieved by increasing the excretion of potassium. This can be done with diuretics that increase potassium excretion through urine. Kayexalate binds with potassium to increase secretion and can be given rectally by enema. This will cause increased excretion of potassium through the GI tract. IV fluids high in glucose concentration can cause potassium to move from the extracellular to the intracellular space.

Hypocalcemia

Hypocalcemia can be caused by under secretion of parathyroid hormone, resulting in more calcium remaining in the bones and less being circulated into the bloodstream. Calcium requires vitamin D to be absorbed in the GI tract, so a vitamin D deficiency can lead to hypocalcemia. This can also result from an alteration in renal function.

With hypocalcemia there is excitability of the nervous system. Patients may exhibit spasm of the facial muscles (a positive Chvostek's sign). Mental status will be altered, and patients may even experience hallucinations. The heart rate may become irregular, and changes may be present on EKG. Muscle spasms can occur in the smooth muscle, such as the bronchial passages, leading to respiratory arrest.

Treatment can be with calcium replacement if calcium levels have dropped dangerously low. Serum calcium values should be monitored regularly to assess for resolution of the condition and to detect if the calcium levels are decreasing further. Seizures precautions may be necessary if patients develop alterations in motor activity.

Hypercalcemia

Hypercalcemia is an increased level of calcium in the serum, >10.5. Calcium levels within the bloodstream are controlled by many factors, one of which is parathyroid hormone. This causes calcium to be reabsorbed by the bones if the level is too high or causes it to escape the bones and enter the circulating bloodstream if levels are too low. Any tumors affecting this process can alter calcium levels and cause an elevated calcium level. Calcium is excreted by the renal system, and any alteration in kidney function could result in hypercalcemia. An increase in heart rate can occur. Patients will have changes in mental status with lethargy and somnolence being present. There may be a decrease in the peripheral reflexes because of malfunction in nerve transmissions. Decreased urinary output due to kidney dysfunction may occur.

Treatment is with IV steroids. Gallium nitrate may be used with cancer-induced hypercalcemia. Patients should be encouraged to increase activity levels and perform light exercise as tolerated to build bone density.

Hypomagnesemia

Hypomagnesemia is defined as a serum magnesium level <1.8. Magnesium is stored in the liver, and liver failure can cause the magnesium stores to be depleted. Some antibiotics and diuretics can cause a decrease in magnesium levels. Magnesium is responsible for maintaining normal electrolyte levels within the cells, so changes in sodium and potassium levels may affect magnesium levels. Magnesium has an adverse relationship with calcium levels, so if there is an increase in calcium, there will be a concomitant decrease in magnesium.

Symptoms include changes in mental status and somnolence, decreased reflexes, and/or seizures. Vasodilation may cause erythema and hypotension. There may be a decrease in respiratory rate.

To treat hypomagnesemia, magnesium sulfate can be given. There are also medications that help to decrease the amount of magnesium that is excreted through the renal and urinary systems. Potassium and sodium levels should also be closely monitored to ensure these remain within normal limits.

Metabolic alkalosis

Metabolic alkalosis occurs when the pH of the blood becomes too elevated. This can occur due to a decrease in hydrogen ions or a direct increase in bicarbonate ions. The means by which these two actions occur is usually through the GI tract or through the renal tubule system. With the loss of hydrochloric acid in the stomach, such as with vomiting or NG tube suctioning, an alkalotic state can develop. Renal dysfunction or diuretic use can cause decreased secretion of bicarbonate ions, and this raises the bicarbonate levels.

Symptoms include signs of hypocalcemia (Chvostek's sign, changes in mental status), hypervolemia, and hypertension. Signs of bulimia, such as dental caries and electrolyte abnormalities may be present. Lab studies show an elevated serum pH, elevated bicarbonate levels, and possibly elevated aldosterone levels.

Treatment is with correction of the underlying cause. IV sodium chloride can help to restore the acid-base balance. If edema is present, potassium chloride should be used to balance electrolytes and reduce the edema.

Metabolic acidosis

Metabolic acidosis is a condition in which there are excess hydrogen ions within the system, resulting in a decrease in serum pH levels. This can be due to excessive intake of acidic substances, such as aspirin products, methanol, or antifreeze. Diabetes can also be a cause of metabolic acidosis. Metabolic dysfunction can also cause decreased secretion of hydrogen, leading to retention of more acid than the body needs.

The body will try to compensate for this condition by increasing the respiratory rate and increasing the depth of respirations in an effort to "blow off" some of the excess hydrogen through carbon dioxide. Patients may become stuporous, and death may result without treatment. Lab studies will reveal a decrease in serum pH levels and possibly elevated chloride levels. If diabetes is the cause, glucose levels will often be very high.

Treatment can be accomplished through IV fluids, but if severe, bicarbonate infusions may be necessary. Treating the underlying cause should be the focus of treatment.

Respiratory alkalosis

Respiratory alkalosis usually occurs due to an excessive loss of carbon dioxide through respirations. This can occur with chronic respiratory illnesses or may be acute in nature. When chronic, the body will compensate and adjust to the excess loss of chloride by decreasing excretion of bicarbonate ions through the urine.

Chronic respiratory alkalosis will not cause patients to experience any symptoms. When acute, patients may experience light-headedness, dizziness, paresthesias, and syncope. This can be seen with hyperventilation. On exam, patients may be visibly hyperventilating or short of breath and carpopedal spasms may be present. Fever can raise the respiratory rate and lead to hyperventilation, which can cause respiratory alkalosis.

Treatment is by treating the underlying cause. Frequently, the chronic form of the condition is not treated. With symptomatic respiratory alkalosis, effort should be made to correct the acid-base imbalance by slowing down the respiratory rate and administering oxygen. If fever is the cause, antipyretics should be given and the underlying cause of the fever should be treated.

Respiratory acidosis

Respiratory acidosis is due to a depressed respiratory system that prevents carbon dioxide from being "blown off," leading to elevated acid levels. This can be an acute or chronic condition that may or may not require treatment. Some common causes are primary respiratory illness that causes a depressed respiratory system, CNS dysfunction that affects the respiratory center in the hypothalamus, or unknown cause.

Patients may exhibit a decreased respiratory rate with mental status changes, somnolence, or stupor. If chronic in nature, patients may appear largely asymptomatic. Pulse oximetry will show a decrease in O_2 saturation. If severe, patients may appear cyanotic, especially in the nail beds and circum-orally.

Treatment may not be necessary if this is a chronic condition and patients are not especially symptomatic. Otherwise, the underlying cause should be treated. Medications can be given to make respirations more productive. Mechanical ventilation with intubation may be necessary.

Leiomyoma

Leiomyomas, or uterine fibroids, are very common benign uterine tumors. They usually form during the childbearing years, and most women are not aware they have them because they are frequently asymptomatic. Leiomyomas may be caused by genetic factors or hormones, especially estrogen and progesterone.

Most women are asymptomatic from leiomyomas. When they do produce symptoms, patients will complain of heavy bleeding that may or may not be associated with menstrual periods. Leiomyomas may be large enough to cause abdominal or pelvic pain and pressure. If compressing on the colon, they can cause constipation. If applying pressure to the bladder, they can cause urinary frequency or incontinence.

A hysterectomy can be performed to remove the uterus if the symptoms are severe and the woman is not planning to have any more children. Laser ablation can also be attempted to shrink the tumors. Medications may be tried, such as gonadotropin-releasing hormone agonists or androgen hormones to reduce symptoms.

Hematologic

Vitamin B-12 deficiency

A deficiency in vitamin B12, or pernicious anemia, can occur in those who do not consume enough foods high in B12, such as dairy products and meat. It is most often due to a lack of intrinsic factor in the stomach. This factor is necessary for the absorption of B12. Past surgeries to remove portions of the GI tract can also decrease the absorption of B12.

A deficiency of vitamin B12 can cause chronic fatigue and a loss of appetite. Patients may appear pale and short of breath. Paresthesias may develop in the extremities, and the condition can progress to the point of mental changes, such as confusion.

Treatment is with vitamin B12 replacement. This can be administered by intramuscular injection or nasal spray. Treatment begins with daily doses of the vitamin supplement, but then decreases to once monthly. Vitamin B12 levels should be monitored to measure the effectiveness of treatment.

Sickle cell anemia

Sickle cell anemia is a genetic form of anemia that affects the red blood cells. The cells are crescent-shaped and cannot carry oxygen effectively. This results in a decrease in oxygen being delivered to the tissues. Because of their shape, the cells can become adhered to the wall of small vessels, causing vascular occlusion in the affected area. This condition is more common in African-Americans and Hispanics, and both parents must carry the gene in order for a child to develop the disease.

Patients will be anemic and will have episodes of pain, particularly in the extremities. Swollen hands and feet are common and extreme pain can develop during a sickle cell crisis. Sequestration syndrome can occur in which the organs are affected, especially the spleen.

Treatment is supportive with pain relievers, blood transfusions, and oxygen. Bone marrow transplant may be helpful in curing the disease, but finding a matching donor can be difficult.

Clotting disorders

- Factor VII disorder is due to a lack of extrinsic factor, which is necessary to complete the clotting cascade. A prolonged PT and normal PTT will be present. Treatment is with infusions of plasma, factor VII concentrates, or recombinant factor VII.
- Factor IX disorder is also called hemophilia B. It is a genetic disorder found on the X chromosome so it affects males more than females. A prolonged PTT, normal PT, normal bleeding time, and normal fibrinogen levels will be present. Treatment is with infusions of factor IX.
- Factor XI disorder is also called Rosenthal syndrome or hemophilia C. It occurs in both males and females and is more common in the Jewish population. It is also more common in children with Noonan syndrome. A prolonged PTT and normal PT will be present. Infusions of fresh frozen plasma (FFP) are the primary treatment. Factor XI concentrates are also available for treatment.

Epstein-Barr infection

Most people are carriers of the Epstein-Barr virus, but may not have developed an active infection from the virus. It is a form of herpes virus (human herpes virus 4) and is responsible for causing infectious mononucleosis. It is transmitted through saliva.

Symptoms of an Epstein-Barr infection include swollen painful lymph nodes, extreme fatigue, and sore throat. Fever may also be present. This is most common in teenagers or college-age young adults. The white blood cell count will be elevated with increased lymphocytes in the differential. A Mono Spot test will be positive for infection.

Treatment is supportive, and antibiotics are not helpful in treating this viral infection. Analgesics, increased fluid intake, and rest will help to relieve some of the symptoms. Warm salt water gargles can help with the sore throat. The symptoms of the infection may last for several weeks. A patient will not contract mononucleosis again after the initial exposure to the Epstein-Barr virus.

Infectious Diseases

Pinworm infection

The pinworm is a type of roundworm. The worms will lay eggs within the digestive tract and then they travel to the anal area where they are usually found. Pinworms can be effectively treated, but serious complications can develop if the infestation is severe. Pinworms are more prevalent in warmer areas of the country and infestations occur more frequently in children. Pinworms are highly contagious. As a patient itches the anal area where the eggs are located, the eggs cling to the fingers and can easily be transmitted to other people either directly or through food or surfaces. The eggs can thrive for 2-3 weeks on an inanimate object.

Patients will have anal itching that can be intense. Itching is usually worse at night and can cause insomnia. Abdominal pain, nausea, and vomiting can also occur.

Anti-parasitic medications are given to kill the pinworms and their larvae. The most effective drugs used are Pin-X® and Albenza®. The entire family should be treated because pinworms are so contagious.

Lyme disease

Lyme disease can occur from a bite from an infected deer tick. It is more prevalent in heavily wooded areas. Those who spend time outdoors, especially in wooded areas or tall grass, are more at risk for being bitten from an infected deer tick. Having exposed skin when walking in these types of areas will also increase the risk of developing Lyme disease.

The bite from an infected deer tick will leave an erythematous area on the skin and the tick may still be attached. A few days later, a bull's eye rash can develop that may be small or large. Lyme disease can progress to cause severe joint pain, paresthesias, Bell's palsy, confusion, fatigue, and heart palpitations.

Antibiotic treatment with doxycycline or amoxicillin is started immediately after diagnosis. It may be necessary to treat with IV infusions of antibiotics, depending on the severity of the disease. Supportive therapy with pain relievers may help with the pain associated with Lyme disease.

Syphilis

Syphilis is a bacterial sexually-transmitted disease. It is most common in homosexual men who have unprotected sex. It is caused by the bacteria *Treponema pallidum* and can be transmitted from mother to fetus during pregnancy.

Within a few days of contact, a painless chancre sore will develop where the infection was contracted, usually the genitals. This usually heals without treatment. The next phase of syphilis occurs 2-10 weeks later with the development of a rash characterized by red lesions, about 1-inch in diameter, which can occur anywhere on the body. This rash can also be found on the palms and soles. Patients may also have vague, flu-like symptoms. The final stage of syphilis may occur many years later. This stage includes neurological changes, including meningitis, dementia, or paralysis. Aortic aneurysm and cardiac valve disease can also occur.

Diagnosis is with an RPR blood test, which will be elevated with syphilis infection. Treatment is with penicillin or appropriate antibiotic therapy if patients are penicillin-allergic.

Musculoskeletal

Fractures

Boxer's fracture – This occurs at the distal end of the fifth metacarpal bone. It earned its name because it is usually caused by force of a fist hitting a hard surface, as with boxing. It usually resolves within 4-6 weeks with rest, compression, and elevation. Casting may or may not be necessary depending on the severity of the fracture.

Colles fracture – This occurs at the distal end of the radius. It is usually caused by breaking a fall with an outstretched hand, causing extreme force to be applied to the arm. Depending on severity, a cast is applied for 6 weeks until the fracture has healed. Surgery may be necessary with a displaced fracture.

Scaphoid fracture – This occurs from a fall on an outstretched hand. This will cause tenderness in the anatomic snuffbox at the base of the thumb in the wrist. There is risk of interrupted blood supply to the small bone with this fracture. Treatment is with casting, sometimes up to 10-12 weeks, and surgery may be necessary.

Gamekeeper's thumb

Gamekeeper's thumb, or skier's thumb, is injury to the ulnar collateral ligament of the thumb. It is caused by a force that hyperextends the thumb away from the hand toward the body, as when falling on a ski pole. It earned its name from gamekeepers in Europe injuring the ligament while breaking rabbits' necks.

Patients will have significant pain with this injury and, depending upon severity, it can be disabling. The pain is greatly exacerbated when trying to grasp or pinch anything, like when holding car keys. The area may be edematous, erythematous, or ecchymotic. Exam may reveal ligament instability.

Treatment is with immobilization of the ligament, possibly with casting depending on severity, and pain relievers. Surgery may be necessary if the ligament injury is not healing or if there is a complete non-healing tear. Stretching of the ligament may be necessary following immobilization to regain normal range of motion.

Nursemaid's elbow

Nursemaid's elbow is a subluxation of the radial head. It occurs in children under 6-years-old. A pulling mechanism on the arm, such as when swinging a child, causes the radial head to pull out of the capsule in which it sits. This results in partial dislocation, or subluxation, of the arm.

The child will initially experience pain with this condition. The child may continue to act normally but will refuse to use the affected arm. There is no actual deformity of the arm visible, but the child will guard the arm and prevent any movement of it to prevent pain.

A nursemaid's elbow is easily reduced. The child's arm should be extended, the hand supinated, and then the elbow flexed so the hand touches the shoulder. If this does not reduce the subluxation, the arm may be placed in a sling and orthopedic evaluation obtained to determine whether surgery is warranted. The parents should be advised to avoid swinging or pulling the child to prevent this from happening again.

Carpal tunnel syndrome

Carpal tunnel syndrome occurs when there is irritation and pressure applied to the median nerve within the carpal tunnel of the wrist. It can have no known cause, but most patients have experienced some type of repetitive movement of the hands that caused irritation within the carpal tunnel.
Symptoms will be gradually progressive and include numbness or tingling of the thumb, index, and middle fingers. Symptoms can be elicited by tapping on the inner wrist over the carpal tunnel (Tinel's sign). Symptoms may be worse at night and may wake patients. Patients may describe grip strength weakness and frequent dropping of objects at home. EMG and nerve conduction testing will reveal a diagnosis of carpal tunnel syndrome.

Cock-up wrist splints should be tried to help relieve pressure on the nerve and reduce the symptoms. Anti-inflammatory drugs and resting the hands and wrists may help. Surgery to release the ligament over the carpal tunnel usually resolves the condition.

De Quervain's tenosynovitis

De Quervain's tenosynovitis is a condition in which there is inflammation in the abductor pollicis longus and extensor pollicis brevis tendons in the thumb. They are held together in the thumb by the extensor retinaculum. If the tendons become inflamed and swollen, the retinaculum cannot expand to accommodate the inflammation, leading to tenosynovitis. This can be caused by overuse of the thumbs. The pain is reproducible with moving the thumb away from the palm and backwards. Arthritis and trauma can also cause edema in the tendons, leading to this condition. Pregnancy can cause water retention, which may lead to constriction and pain of the tendons.

Treatment is with rest of the thumbs. Ice can be applied to relieve the pain. Anti-inflammatory drugs may help with pain relief, also. Splints can be applied that restrict the thumb movements and reduce pain. If conservative treatments do not help, steroid injections into the tendons may reduce the inflammation. As a last resort, surgery can be done to release the extensor retinaculum.

Medial epicondylitis

Medial epicondylitis, or golfer's elbow, occurs due to overuse of the flexor muscles in the forearm. These muscles attach to a tendon that attaches to the medial epicondyle of the elbow. With overuse, such as with golfing, inflammation in the tendon can occur.

Patients will complain of pain and tenderness over the medial epicondyle, aggravated by flexing the fingers and wrist. Hand or wrist weakness may develop. All symptoms will become worse while grasping an object. Testing involves having patients extend the palm outward and attempt to flex the wrist toward the arm against pressure. This will reproduce the pain.

Treatment is rest of the elbow and forearm. A splint can be worn at the elbow to relieve pain and ice can be applied. Anti-inflammatory drugs may also help. Steroid injections can be performed in the tendon at the medial epicondyle. Exercises can be done, also, to help strengthen the flexor muscles of the forearm.

Lateral epicondylitis

Lateral epicondylitis, or tennis elbow, occurs due to overuse of the extensor muscles in the forearm. These muscles attach to a tendon that attaches to the lateral epicondyle of the elbow. With overuse, such as with playing tennis, inflammation in the tendon can occur.

Patients will complain of pain and tenderness over the lateral epicondyle, aggravated with extending the fingers and wrist. Hand or wrist weakness may develop. All symptoms will become worse while picking up an object. Testing involves having patients extend the wrist or fingers against resistance. This will reproduce the pain.

Treatment is with rest of the elbow and forearm. A splint can be worn at the elbow to relieve pain and ice can be applied. Anti-inflammatory drugs may also help. Steroid injections can be performed in the tendon at the lateral epicondyle. Exercises can be done, also, to help strengthen the extensor muscles of the forearm.

Ankylosing spondylitis

Ankylosing spondylitis is an inflammatory form of arthritis that can affect any of the joints in the body. It most commonly affects the joints in the vertebral column and the sacroiliac joints. The inflammation that occurs causes bony overgrowth, especially in the spine, and leads to fusion of the vertebral bodies. When it occurs at the joints of the ribs and spine, rib cage mobility can be affected, restricting respirations. Patients will complain of pain and stiffness in the affected joints. This will lead to a stooped posture and possibly depressed respirations. Iritis and inflammatory bowel disease is also common with ankylosing spondylitis. X-rays will show the bony fusion that occurs, especially in the vertebral column. Blood testing includes CRP, ESR, and CBC to check for inflammation. Genetic testing for the HLA-B27 gene indicates a person's predilection for developing this condition.

Treatment is with pain relievers and anti-inflammatory drugs. Steroids may be necessary to decrease inflammation. Infusions of Embral® or Remicade® may also help to decrease symptoms.

Cauda equina syndrome

Cauda equina syndrome is a condition in which there is severe compression of the nerve roots exiting the spinal canal from the cauda equina below the termination of the spinal cord at L1. It is usually caused by an acute herniated nucleus pulposus (herniated disc) or can occur due to progressive degenerative changes causing severe spinal stenosis in the lower lumbar spine.

Patients will usually have low back pain with pain radiating into one or both of the lower extremities. There will be saddle anesthesia present along with bowel and bladder incontinence. The lower extremities will be numb and/or weak. There will also be depressed or absent reflexes in the lower extremities.

Steroids can be started to reduce the inflammation, but this is usually only until surgery is performed. Treatment of cauda equina syndrome is urgent surgical intervention. If treated promptly, there is a chance that patients' symptoms will be reversed. The longer the symptoms are present, however, the less likely patients will reach a full recovery.

Herniated nucleus pulposus

A herniated nucleus pulposus, or herniated disc, can occur anywhere in the spinal column. The disc can bulge in one direction of may be central. If this occurs above the level of L1, there is a risk of spinal cord compression.

Patients will complain of pain at the level of the spine where the herniation occurs, along with radicular pain following the dermatome of the affected nerve. For example, if the herniation occurs at L5-S1, patients may complain of sciatic-type pain. Patients may develop numbness or tingling in the affected dermatome, along with weakness of the affected limb.

Patients should be started on anti-inflammatory drugs and pain relievers. Often, the symptoms will resolve with conservative treatment. Physical therapy to help with pain relief and stretching and strengthening can help. Steroids, either orally or per epidural injection, can help to reduce the inflammation. Surgery can also be done with a microdiskectomy to remove the portion of the disc that has herniated.

Spinal stenosis

Spinal stenosis occurs when there is disc or bony material, causing narrowing of the spinal canal. In the upper spine, this can cause compression of the spinal cord, and in the lower lumbar spine it will cause compression on the nerves of the cauda equina. Spinal stenosis is most often degenerative in nature. It can also occur with traumatic disc herniation or spondylolisthesis. Patients will complain of pain in the affected portion of the spine with pain, numbness, and/or weakness extending into the upper or lower extremities, depending on location. With spinal cord stenosis, there will be profound weakness and hyperactive reflexes/spasticity. Symptoms of neurogenic claudication are due to lumbar spinal stenosis and include pain that is aggravated with walking and standing. These are usually somewhat relieved with sitting and leaning forward.

Symptoms may be slightly relieved with anti-inflammatory drugs and pain relievers. Surgical correction can be performed with a laminectomy or X-Stop procedure that relieves the pressure being applied to the spinal canal.

Avascular necrosis

Avascular necrosis usually affects the upper femur at the hip but can occur in other bones as well. It occurs when there is a loss of blood supply to the bone. Chronic steroid use can cause this condition, as can radiation treatments to the area or chemotherapy. Alcoholism can lead to occlusion of the vessels providing blood to the bones and may lead to avascular necrosis. Chronic medical conditions, such as sickle cell anemia and lupus, may also cause this condition.

Pain is the most common symptom of avascular necrosis. Patients may have noticed a gradual progression of the pain or may develop a pathologic fracture. X-rays will show the dead bone tissue once the condition is advanced. MRI is more sensitive in detecting early disease.

Treatment should focus on treating the underlying cause and restoring blood supply to the bone. Joint replacement or bone grafting may be necessary. A core decompression procedure can remove the inner layer of bone to help regenerate the blood vessels, restoring blood supply.

Slipped capital femoral epiphysis

A slipped capital femoral epiphysis is a condition in which the proximal femoral growth plate becomes unstable. This can occur because of trauma causing a Salter-Harris fracture, obesity, or abnormal growth of the bone and cartilage in the growth plate itself. It is most commonly detected in children from 10-16 years of age. It usually occurs unilaterally, but may occur bilaterally, especially in children under the age of 10.

Patients will develop a limp that becomes progressively worse. They will complain of pain in the hip, groin, thigh, or even in the knee. X-rays will show displacement of the femoral head, from mild to severe.

Surgical repair is necessary to correct this condition. An open reduction and internal fixation of the femoral head is performed to stabilize the joint. With severe disease, the child may end up with a discrepancy in the leg lengths, which can lead to chronic limp.

Osgood-Schlatter disease

Osgood-Schlatter disease is a condition in which inflammation develops around the tibial tuberosity at the knee. It occurs with repeated stress on the patellar tendon, such as with running and kicking, and can cause the tendon to slightly pull away at its attachment to the tibial tuberosity. In severe cases, the tendon can completely tear at its attachment point. This is most common in active children, usually in their early teens, involved in sports.

Patients will complain of pain in the knee at the tibial tuberosity. There may be swelling, redness, and decreased motion of the knee present. The pain is aggravated with running, kicking, and squatting.

Rest will usually resolve the condition. Mild analgesics, NSAIDs, and ice can also help to relieve the pain. This condition can last for weeks to months, so it can be frustrating to the child to limit sports activities. Rarely, surgery is necessary if the tendon has torn and is not healing on its own.

Septic arthritis

Septic arthritis is an infection in a joint, most commonly the knee though other joints may be affected. This is usually due to a bacterial infection that has spread to the joint, but it can be caused by fungus also. The most common bacterial causes are *Staphylococcus aureus* or *Neisseria gonorrhea*.

Patients will complain of significant pain in the affected joint with fever and chills. They may have some nausea and vomiting. They may or may not be aware of a recent bacterial infection elsewhere in their body. The joint will appear red, swollen, hot, and very tender to the touch. Aspiration of the infectious material in the knee will show purulent discharge, possibly with some blood present. Culture and sensitivity testing of the infectious material should be performed.

Treatment is with IV antibiotics started at the time of diagnosis. This will be followed by a course of oral antibiotics. If the condition is severe, surgery may be necessary to flush the joint to remove the infectious material.

Ganglion cyst

A ganglion cyst is a benign cyst that most commonly forms in the wrists or hands. It can also occur in the feet. There is no known cause for cyst formation, but the tissue surrounding a tendon may bulge, causing synovial fluid to accumulate within it. Patients will notice the cyst on the wrist or hand. It is usually not a painful condition though, if it becomes large enough, it can cause nerve compression, which leads to pain, numbness, or weakness in the hands. The symptoms may be similar to those of carpal tunnel syndrome or ulnar neuropathy.

Treatment can begin conservatively with rest of the affected joint to help shrink the cyst. If this does not help, the fluid can be aspirated from the cyst and steroids injected to prevent recurrence. There is a chance the cyst will form again, though. If the cyst causes severe symptoms, surgery can be performed to remove the cyst and decrease the chance of recurrence.

Osteosarcoma

Osteosarcoma is a type of bone cancer that occurs in bones as they are growing. It commonly affects children and young adults from 10-20 years of age. Some hereditary diseases, such as hereditary retinoblastoma, may make children more susceptible to developing bone cancer. Exposure of the bone to high doses of radiation can also increase the risk of this disease. Oftentimes, osteosarcoma will occur without any known cause. Patients will complain of bone pain and may not be diagnosed until they suffer a pathologic fracture. There may be swelling at the site of the cancer. Patients will be fatigued and may or may not have a fever.

The most common treatment for osteosarcoma is surgery to remove the affected portion of the bone. Chemotherapy may be necessary before surgery to shrink the tumor, and it may be used again after surgery. Radiation therapy may also be used to help destroy the cancer cells. In some cases, the cancer can spread to other organs of the body.

Osteoarthritis

Osteoarthritis is a very common condition that occurs due to overuse of the joints. It is characterized by a wearing down of the cartilage within the joints and is a gradually progressive condition. The cause of the condition is use of the joints, especially overuse, and it commonly occurs in the large joints, such as the hips and knees. It can affect any joint in the body. Patients will complain of pain in the affected joint, especially with activity. There may be swelling in the joint. On exam, crepitus can be felt with flexion and extension of the joint. X-rays will show joint space narrowing because of the worn down cartilage.

Treatment is with anti-inflammatory drugs and rest of the affected joint when it is painful. Exercise should still be performed but not to the point that pain occurs. Physical therapy may help with muscle strengthening, and exercises that decrease the stress on joints can be helpful. When osteoarthritis is severe, surgery may be necessary to replace the joint.

Osteoporosis

Osteoporosis is a condition in which there is a decrease in the bone mineral density. It is more common in women than men and is usually post-menopausal. Estrogen is thought to be bone-protective and, with the decrease in estrogen levels after menopause, the bones may begin to weaken. Medications, such as chronic steroid use, can also contribute to the loss of bone density. Smokers and those with a hormonal imbalance, such as hyperparathyroidism, are also more susceptible to developing osteoporosis. Patients may suffer an osteoporotic fracture, such as a compression fracture, as a result of little or no trauma. A DEXA bone density scan will show a bone density of at least 2.5 standard deviations below the value for peak bone mass.

Treatment is with weight-bearing exercise, calcium and vitamin D supplementation, or bisphosphonates or other newer medications that promote absorption of calcium by the bones. If possible, glucocorticoids should be weaned if they are the cause of osteoporosis.

Fibromyalgia

Fibromyalgia is a condition in which patients feels fatigued and has pain "all over." This condition affects the muscles and joints and is diagnosed when no other cause of the symptoms can be found. There is no known cause of fibromyalgia, but it is believed to be a condition in which the body's nervous system becomes hypersensitive to painful stimuli, leading to over activity of the pain receptors in the body. Patients will complain of chronic fatigue accompanied with pain that affects almost the whole body. Signs of depression may also be present. Many patients with fibromyalgia will also suffer from irritable bowel syndrome and chronic headaches.

Treatment is with anti-inflammatory drugs. Narcotic analgesics have not proven to be effective in treating this condition. Current treatment guidelines recommend an SSRI antidepressant to help relieve patients' symptoms. Lyrica® (pregabalin) is an anti-seizure medication that is the first drug indicated for the treatment of fibromyalgia, and it may help relieve the symptoms.

Gout

Gout occurs when there is an accumulation of uric acid in the blood, leading to urate crystals settling in a joint. Gout can be due to excess consumption of foods that are high in uric acid, or can be due to decreased excretion of uric acid by the kidneys. It usually affects the big toe joint but can occur in other joints. It is more common in men than women.

Patients will complain of a sudden onset of severe pain in the affected joint. Even light pressure on the joint causes significant pain. The joint will appear red and swollen and will be very tender when examined.

Treatment is with rest of the affected joint and NSAIDs to decrease the inflammation. Colchicine may be given during an acute attack if it is tolerated. Allopurinol can be taken on a regular basis for prevention of acute episodes for those with chronic gout. Allopurinol increases excretion of uric acid. Patients should also be counseled on dietary changes to decrease their intake of foods high in uric acid.

Pseudogout

Pseudogout is very similar to gout, except the causative agent is different. With pseudogout, the pain and inflammation is due to deposition of calcium pyrophosphate dihydrate crystals within a joint. The most common joints affected by pseudogout are the knees, but it can also occur in the other large joints of the body.

Patients will complain of a sudden onset of severe pain in the affected joint. Even light pressure on the joint causes significant pain. The joint will appear red and swollen and will be very tender when examined.

Treatment is with NSAIDs to reduce the inflammation in the affected joint. Colchicine may be effective in helping to reduce the symptoms, though it can cause several gastrointestinal side effects and may not be well tolerated. Maintenance therapy with colchicine can also be prescribed to help reduce the number of acute attacks of pseudogout. Aspiration of the joint fluid can be performed to relieve pressure on the joint and help to decrease pain.

Polyarteritis nodosa

Polyarteritis nodosa is an autoimmune condition in which inflammation occurs within the arteries. It can occur anywhere within the body, but it most often affects the kidneys, intestines, muscles, and joints. It has no known definite cause, but it is often seen in patients who have been diagnosed with hepatitis B. Patients will complain of pain in the area of the body that is affected by the arterial inflammation. Abdominal pain with bowel involvement, weight loss, and fever are common symptoms. If the inflammation is severe, there can be ischemia of the bowel, kidney, or other affected organs.

Treatment is with high doses of anti-inflammatory drugs, oral and/or IV, such as prednisone or Cytoxan®. Immunosuppressant drugs, such as Imuran®, can be helpful. If patients have hepatitis B, appropriate therapy should be started to treat this condition. If polyarteritis nodosa is severe and tissue death has occurred, surgery may be necessary to remove the ischemic tissue.

Polymyositis

Polymyositis is a connective tissue disease in which inflammation occurs in the muscles. It most commonly affects the muscles in the proximal large joints, such as shoulders and hips, and is gradually progressive in onset. A definite cause is not known, but it may be due to an autoimmune reaction. Patients will complain of a slow progression of muscle weakness and pain. This will commonly be present in the shoulders and arms, and patients will experience a sensation of fatigue after even light activity. They may have some dysphagia that has been progressive, also.

The most common treatments for polymyositis are high dose anti-inflammatory drugs, including steroids, along with physical therapy. There are some experimental medications available that work by suppressing the immune system, but most of them are only available through clinical trials. Complications of polymyositis include possible pneumonia due to decreased chest wall muscle expansion or aspiration pneumonia due to dysphagia.

Polymyalgia rheumatica

Polymyalgia rheumatica is a condition in which patients experience muscle stiffness and aching throughout their bodies. Polymyalgia rheumatica can be insidious in onset or occur very quickly. It is more common in adults over the age of 50, and it may resolve after 1 or 2 years. Polymyalgia rheumatica is an autoimmune disorder, and it is not known exactly what triggers this disease to occur. Patients will complain of muscle pain and stiffness in various locations of the body. As the disease progresses, it will affect both sides equally but may begin in a unilateral distribution. Patients may have a generalized feeling of weakness or malaise, fever, weight loss, and fatigue. Anemia of chronic disease can also develop in time.

Treatment of the muscle pain is attempted with NSAIDs. Treatment with corticosteroids may be necessary as symptoms become debilitating. Patients should be counseled on the risks of long-term steroid use and should be closely monitored.

Reiter's syndrome

Reiter's syndrome is a collection of three syndromes: arthritis, redness of the eyes, and urinary tract symptoms. This condition is also called reactive arthritis because it can occur in response to an infection somewhere in the body. The most common predisposing infection is *Chlamydia.* and symptoms of Reiter's usually appear 1-3 weeks following infection. Other less common bacteria that may cause Reiter's syndrome include *Salmonella* and *Shigella.* It is more common in young adult males.

The arthritis primarily affects the joints in the lower extremities and spine. Sacroiliitis and spondylitis of the spine are common. Conjunctivitis and uveitis also usually occur, and these symptoms may wax and wane during the course of the illness. Patients will have complaints of dysuria, urinary frequency, discharge, and prostatitis in men.

Symptomatic treatment is indicated for Reiter's syndrome. If there is an active infection, appropriate antibiotics should be given. NSAIDs and corticosteroids can be helpful.

Rheumatoid arthritis

Rheumatoid arthritis is a progressive disease that affects the synovial linings of the joints. The body's white blood cells attack this synovial lining and destroy it, leading to deformity and destruction of the joint. It is usually diagnosed in middle age and is more likely to occur in females than males. Patients will have a gradual progression of joint pain that generally starts in the small joints of the hands, wrists, ankles, and feet first. It will eventually spread to include the larger joints of the body. They will notice swelling and possibly redness of the joints, along with decreased movement as the disease progresses.

There is no cure for rheumatoid arthritis, but symptoms can be controlled. NSAIDs and pain medications can help with pain relief. Immunosuppressants, such as Imuran®, and TNF-alpha suppressants, such as

Enbrel®, can help to prevent flare-ups of the condition and control symptoms. In severe cases, joint replacement surgery may be necessary.

Systemic lupus erythematous

Lupus is a condition in which the body's immune system turns against itself and begins attacking organs, tissues, and blood cells. There is no definite known cause of lupus, but it is thought that genetic factors may play a part in developing the disease. There may be some influence from environmental factors as well.

The malar rash (butterfly) across the nose and cheeks is common with lupus, and patients may complain of other skin lesions that come and go. Joint pain and stiffness is common, as is Raynaud's phenomenon. Patients may have chronic fatigue and weakness, along with depression.

There is no known cure for lupus, but the symptoms can usually be controlled. NSAIDs and corticosteroids can help to decrease inflammation during an acute flare-up. Some of the symptoms of lupus respond to anti-malarial drugs though it is not known why. Immunosuppressant medications may also be helpful in decreasing the symptoms of lupus.

Sjögren's syndrome

Sjögren's syndrome is an autoimmune disorder that is often seen with other types of connective tissue disorders. It is not known what causes Sjögren's syndrome though it is suspected that hereditary factors may play a part. There may also be a link with a bacterial or viral infection. Sjögren's syndrome is more common in women than men. The primary symptoms seen with Sjögren's are dry eyes and a dry mouth. Rarely, it can cause lung, kidney, or liver damage. Since it is commonly seen in conjunction with other connective tissue disorders, symptoms of those accompanying diseases may also be present.

There are medications that can help specifically with the dry eyes and dry mouth associated with Sjögren's syndrome. Systemic medications to treat the symptoms include corticosteroids and immunosuppressants, especially if another connective tissue disorder is present. If dry eyes are severe, surgery can be performed to block small openings in the eyelids that drain tears from the eyes, thereby retaining moisture within the eyes.

Scleroderma

Scleroderma is a condition in which hardening of the skin and connective tissues occur. This can become progressively worse and lead to involvement of the organs. There is no definite known cause of scleroderma, but it is an autoimmune connective tissue disorder. It is more common in women than men.

Patients will complain of some areas of thickened or hardened skin that will not go away. As the condition progresses, the skin becomes stiffer and range of motion of the limbs is decreased. Scleroderma can even affect the organs, such as the stomach, and lead to decreased gastric motility. It can also affect the kidneys, and when severe, result in renal failure.

Topical medications can be used to help decrease inflammation over the thickened areas of skin. NSAIDs and corticosteroids can help with pain as stiffness occurs. Medications to improve circulation can help, as can immunosuppressants to decrease the symptoms and progression of scleroderma.

Neurologic System

Cerebral palsy

Cerebral palsy is a condition that develops due to brain damage during development. It affects a child's motor development and may or may not be accompanied by mental retardation. Cerebral palsy affects motor function by causing the muscles to be flaccid and weak or rigid and spastic. It can be caused by infections in the mother during pregnancy or improper brain development after birth.

Parents will notice their children are not reaching developmental milestones, like sitting up, crawling, or walking, as they should. The limbs will appear under-developed and flaccid or, more commonly, stiff and rigid. The child will be uncoordinated and hyper-reflexic. There is no cure for cerebral palsy. Physical therapy and kinesiotherapy can help with stretching the muscles and preventing contractions due to rigidity. Muscle relaxants can also be given to help decrease rigidity in the limbs. If there are learning impairments, special education should be utilized to maximize the child's learning potential.

Bell's palsy

Bell's palsy is a condition in which the seventh cranial nerve, the facial nerve, is weakened or paralyzed. It can be caused by a viral infection, pregnancy, or an autoimmune condition. Patients will notice a rather rapid onset of weakness on one side of the face. This can occur quite suddenly or may come on gradually over the course of a couple of days. There will be difficulty closing the eye on the affected side, smiling, or clenching teeth, and a headache may be present. Some patients may experience pain in front of the ear on the affected side, usually a couple of days before the palsy sets in.

Bell's palsy is almost always a self-limiting condition that last from a week to a few months. Giving corticosteroids early on may help reduce the symptoms and reduce inflammation surrounding the facial nerve. Antiviral medications may be helpful in reducing symptoms. Lubricating eye drops may be helpful with dry eye on the affected side.

Guillain-Barré syndrome

Guillain-Barré is a condition in which inflammation occurs in the nerves throughout the body, resulting in muscle weakness and occasionally respiratory depression. There is no definite known cause of this disease, but over one-half of the people who suffer from Guillain-Barré have a history of a respiratory or gastrointestinal illness before they develop symptoms. It may be due to an autoimmune disorder. Patients will develop weakness and numbness in the extremities that gradually spreads up the limbs. Depending on the severity of the illness, patients may have paralysis of the diaphragm that requires mechanical ventilation. This can be accompanied with hypotension and bladder/bowel incontinence.

Plasmapheresis can help to remove antibodies that may contribute to the symptoms of Guillain-Barré. Alternately, immunoglobulin intravenously can help decrease symptoms. The disorder generally begins to resolve after approximately 1 month. Most people make a full recovery from Guillain-Barré with a small portion of patients having some degree of residual weakness.

Myasthenia gravis

Myasthenia gravis is a neurologic disorder that causes muscle fatigue with activity. It is an autoimmune disorder in which the body blocks the acetylcholine receptor sites at the neuromuscular junction. This leads to fewer nerve signals being sent to the muscle cells, resulting in weakness. It most commonly affects middle-aged men and women. There is no definite known cause of myasthenia gravis, but the thymus gland may play a role in producing the antibodies for the disease. Patients will complain of weakness with any activity, relieved with rest. They may have trouble with their eyelids drooping and difficulty chewing or swallowing. When severe, myasthenia gravis can even affect normal respirations. Diagnosis is by injecting Tensilon and monitoring for an improvement in symptoms.

There is no cure for myasthenia gravis, but symptoms can be controlled with immunosuppressant medications. Plasmapheresis and immunoglobulin infusions may also help in reducing the symptoms. A small percentage of patients will improve after removal of the thymus gland.

Cluster headaches

Cluster headaches are characterized by periods when headaches will happen frequently, perhaps for a few days or months, and then go into remission without headaches for a period of time. There is no definite known cause of cluster headaches though it has been found that they are more common in males who are heavy drinkers and smokers. Dysfunction of the hypothalamus gland may also play a role.

Cluster headaches are very severe and are more likely to occur at night. Patients will not usually have an aura or triggering event for the headache. They will describe a nasal congestion at the time of the headache, possibly with swelling around the eyes.

Administering oxygen during a cluster headache can help decrease the severity and length of the headache. Imitrex® injections can also help at the beginning of the headache. Some patients respond well to dihydroergotamine or local anesthetics administered nasally.

Migraine headaches

Migraine headaches are fairly common and occur more in women than men. It is thought that there are several factors that may trigger a migraine. Changes in hormone levels during the menstrual cycle may trigger these, as can certain foods such as alcohol, chocolate, fermented or pickled foods, and caffeine. Stress and changes in the environment may trigger a migraine. Patients may or may not describe an aura before the headache begins. This can include a tingling sensation, change in smell or taste, or visual changes. The headache is severe and usually affects one side of the head. It may be accompanied by photophobia, phonophobia, or nausea and vomiting.

Treatment with triptan medications at the first sign of a migraine can help to abort it or decrease the intensity of the pain. Pain relievers, ergot medications, and anti-emetics can also help. Prophylactic medication, such as beta-blockers, can also help to decrease the incidence of migraines.

Tension headaches

Tension headaches are the most common type of headache, and just about everyone has had one at some point in his/her life. It is thought headaches may be due to many factors. Changes in the balance of neurotransmitters within the brain may contribute as can fluctuating hormone levels. Increased alcohol, caffeine, or tobacco use may also cause tension headaches. Daily stress, lack of sleep, or missing a meal can also contribute to tension headaches. Patients will describe headache pain that usually feels like a band around the skull. It may affect the whole head or only one side. The headache can radiate down to the neck and cause neck and upper back pain. Rarely will people have nausea or vomiting with tension headaches.

Decreasing stress and other lifestyle changes can help control chronic tension headaches. Avoiding alcohol and caffeine and quitting smoking can also help. NSAIDs and other pain relievers may help, but with excessive use, NSAIDs can contribute to rebound headaches.

Encephalitis

Encephalitis is a viral infection of the brain that can be primary or can occur due to a viral infection elsewhere in the body. The most common viruses to cause this are the herpes virus, especially herpes simplex, Epstein-Barr, and varicella-zoster. Arboviruses can cause encephalitis, such as Eastern and Western equine encephalitis or West Nile encephalitis. Patients may have few symptoms, or the disease may be severe. They may complain of a severe headache accompanied by nausea and vomiting. Visual changes may occur and seizures may be present. If encephalitis is severe, mental confusion and lethargy may be present.

Treatment is mainly supportive. NSAIDs can help reduce the inflammation around the brain and narcotics can help with the pain. Anticonvulsants may be necessary if patients are having seizures. If a herpes virus is the causative organism, acyclovir may help to reduce symptoms and shorten the length of the illness. Research is being done on interferon as an immunosuppressant therapy to treat encephalitis.

Meningitis

Meningitis is an infection of the meninges that surround the brain and spinal cord. It is most often due to a virus and is self-limiting, but it can be fatal if a bacterium is the cause. The most common cause of bacterial meningitis is *Streptococcus pneumoniae*, with *Neisseria meningitides* as the second leading cause. *H. influenzae* and *Listeria monocytogenes* may also cause meningitis. Rarely, fungus can cause the disease. Patients will have a severe headache followed by lethargy and possibly seizures. They may describe neck pain and have neck rigidity on exam. A high fever is usually present along with photophobia. Diagnosis is by lumbar puncture and evaluation of CSF with gram stain and culture and sensitivity. While waiting for lab results to return, IV antibiotics should be started immediately. If the infection is thought to be viral in nature, supportive treatment is all that is necessary, and the illness will usually resolve within 10 days. Bacterial meningitis can be fatal and lead to multi-system organ failure.

Essential tremors

Essential tremors occur in older adults and usually affect the hands though occasionally they can be evident in the legs or even voice. They are not accompanied by any other symptoms, as seen with the tremor of Parkinson's disease, but can be debilitating if severe. Some patients have a genetic predisposition to developing essential tremors, but it is not known what causes the tremors in those who do not have a family history.

Patients will complain of gradually progressive tremors in the hands or other areas. Tremors are most pronounced when performing simple activities, such as eating and drinking, and writing. The tremors usually stop when patients are resting and not moving but restart when they perform activities.

Medications, such as beta-blockers and anticonvulsants, can help control the tremor in most patients. When the tremor is severe and not responding to medical management, a deep brain stimulator can be surgically implanted to try to control the tremor.

Huntington's disease

Huntington's disease is a hereditary disorder of the neurological system. It causes destruction of brain cells and is progressive. It is an autosomal dominant disorder, which means only one parent needs to carry the gene for a child to develop the disease. Early symptoms include personality changes, impaired cognition, and depression. Physical signs include imbalance, uncontrollable facial expressions, lack of coordination, and sudden spasm-like movements. These symptoms gradually progress to the point where patients are incapacitated and cannot care for themselves.

There is no cure for Huntington's disease and patients have a 10-30 year life expectancy after the onset of symptoms. Anticonvulsants, antipsychotics, and antidepressants can help with some of the symptoms. Physical therapy, occupational therapy, and kinesiotherapy can all help with maintaining range of motion and controlled movements of the limbs but will not be able to completely stop the progression of the disease.

Parkinson's disease

Parkinson's disease involves damage or destruction of the neurons that produce the neurotransmitter dopamine in the brain. Dopamine is responsible for allowing the body to move smoothly, without rigidity or jerkiness. The exact cause of Parkinson's is not clearly understood, though it is known that there are genetic tendencies with the disease as well as an increased incidence in people with chronic exposure to herbicides and pesticides.

Symptoms usually occur after the age of 60 but may begin earlier. Patients will develop a shuffling gait, a tremor that may become severe, slowed movements, a flat affect, and sometimes dementia. It can affect speech and swallowing, and some patients may describe a loss of balance.

Treatment is started with levodopa, which is converted to dopamine within the brain. It is frequently given with carbidopa, which increases its concentration within the brain. Other dopamine-agonist medications are also available to increase the dopamine levels within the brain. Surgically, a deep brain stimulator may help with movement disorders associated with Parkinson's.

Generalized convulsive disorder

A generalized convulsive disorder occurs due to an abnormality in the electrical signals in the brain. Researchers believe a genetic abnormality causes a defect in these brain cells. Brain trauma, disease, or a stroke may also increase the chances of developing a convulsive disorder.

Seizures associated with a generalized convulsive disorder may vary. The most mild of these would be a petit mal, or absence seizure, in which patients stare blankly or have very subtle movements. The other end of the spectrum is a grand mal, or tonic-clonic seizure, in which there is a loss of consciousness with generalized jerking and possibly loss of bowel or bladder control.

Treatment is with anticonvulsants, but it may take several trials of drugs to find the most effective treatment for patients. Sometimes multiple medications are necessary. Rarely, surgery can be done if the seizure activity is arising from the frontal lobe of the brain. This procedure involves removing the small portion of the brain in which the seizures are originating.

Generalized nonconvulsive disorder

A generalized nonconvulsive disorder occurs due to an abnormality in the electrical signals in the brain. Researchers believe a genetic abnormality causes a defect in these brain cells. Brain trauma, disease, or a stroke may also increase the chances of developing a nonconvulsive disorder.

This disorder causes partial seizures. Simple partial seizures do not cause a loss of awareness, but rather a change in how things appear, taste, or smell. Patients do not have a change in motor activity with partial seizures. Complex partial seizures will cause a change in consciousness or loss of awareness with some motor changes, such as arm movements, lip smacking, repeated swallowing, or yelling out.
Treatment is with anticonvulsants, but it may take several trials of drugs to find the most effective treatment for patients. Rarely, surgery can be done if the nonconvulsive seizure activity is arising from the frontal lobe of the brain. This involves removing the small portion of the brain in which the seizures are originating.

Status epilepticus

Status epilepticus is a condition in which tonic-clonic or grand mal seizures occur and do not stop. It is considered a medical emergency because of the risk of asphyxiation or respiratory arrest during the seizure. Status epilepticus is most often due to patients not taking the seizure medications correctly but can also occur in acute illnesses such as meningitis, encephalitis, decreased glucose levels, or very high fever.

Patients will exhibit signs of a grand mal seizure persisting after 3 minutes. There may be a known diagnosis of epilepsy or other illness. The airway of patients should be protected and intubation may be necessary. Anticonvulsants are given IV, and Valium is often the treatment of choice to stop the seizure. If the cause of the seizure is not immediately known, an EEG and other testing should be done. If an acute illness is suspected, a lumbar puncture should be done for CSF analysis. Blood cultures should also be drawn to assess for sepsis.

Transient ischemic attack

A transient ischemic attack (TIA), or "mini-stroke," occurs because of atherosclerosis in the brain's arteries. This buildup of cholesterol, or plaque, causes a temporary decrease in oxygen to a certain portion of the brain. About one-third of patients who have a TIA will eventually have a stroke, with most of those occurring within the next year. Patients will have symptoms similar to a stroke with possible hemiparesis, garbled speech, dizziness, and possible loss of vision in one eye. The difference between a stroke and a TIA is that, with a TIA, the symptoms will resolve spontaneously within 24 hours. There are no residual effects from a TIA.

Patients who have had a TIA should be started on anticoagulant or antiplatelet medications. Low-dose aspirin should be given daily. Medications such as Plavix® or Aggrenox® help to prevent platelet aggregation but do not require routine lab work for monitoring like Coumadin®. Lifestyle changes should be implemented, including eating foods lower in fat and cholesterol, quitting smoking, and losing weight if necessary.

Psychiatry/Behavioral

Panic disorder

Panic disorder is a condition in which people experience extreme anxiety that may become severe enough to affect their lives and level of functioning. Panic disorder is characterized by panic attacks that may vary in intensity and frequency and usually occur in young adults. It is twice as likely to affect females. There have been links to panic disorder and exposure to trauma, substance abuse, family history, stress, and defects within the limbic system of the brain.

Panic attacks experienced with panic disorder give patients a sense of extreme anxiety with rapid heartbeat, sweating, dyspnea, shaking, and dizziness. Patients may have a fear of leaving their homes or encountering crowds of people (agoraphobia), or panic disorder may be limited to feelings of anxiety during stressful situations.

Treatment is with behavioral therapies to "talk themselves down" from developing a panic attack. Antidepressant therapy with SSRIs and anti-anxiety medications, such as benzodiazepines, can be helpful. Sensitization therapy with small doses of exposure to the anxiety-provoking stimulus can also be helpful.

Generalized anxiety disorder

Generalized anxiety disorder, or GAD, is a condition in which a person worries all the time about situations or conditions. This worry or stress is out of proportion with the general reaction of most people. It is thought that an imbalance in the neurotransmitters serotonin and norepinephrine may play a role in the development of GAD. GAD causes a generalized state of unrest with muscle tension, irritability, impatience, difficulty concentrating, and insomnia. People may appear very restless with shortness of breath, and they may complain of somatic symptoms such as nausea, diarrhea, or headache.

Psychotherapy can be helpful for the treatment of GAD by having patients develop better coping skills and relaxation methods. Medical treatment is with benzodiazepines for anti-anxiety, such as Xanax® or Ativan®. SSRIs can also control symptoms. Prozac®, Effexor®, and Paxil® have been helpful in treating generalized anxiety disorder. Medical treatment may involve several trials of different medications to find the treatment that works best for patients.

Posttraumatic stress disorder

Posttraumatic stress disorder (PTSD) occurs following involvement in or witness to an extremely traumatic event. This can occur after abuse, from violence to patients or others, or from experiencing a natural disaster. The exact reason some people suffer from PTSD and others do not is not clearly understood.

Symptoms of PTSD usually begin within 3 months of the triggering event but may occur up to years later. Patients will have flashbacks of the trauma, nightmares, irritability, anger, guilt, and possibly substance abuse. They may have difficulty in interpersonal relationships and anhedonia (inability to experience pleasure). Small reminders of the trauma can send them into an episode of anger or fear.

Psychotherapy can be helpful in working through the guilt that may be experienced with PTSD. Developing coping skills to reduce anger that is triggered by reminders of the trauma can also be helpful. Medical treatment varies, depending on the predominant symptoms patients are experiencing. SSRIs and anti-anxiety medications are usually the mainstays of treatment.

Eating disorders

Anorexia nervosa

Anorexia nervosa is an unhealthy obsession with body weight and shape. Patients avoid eating, or will only eat small amounts, to become as thin as possible. Anorexia is caused by an altered perception of body image along with underlying depression. There is often an obsession with perfection. The cause is not clearly understood, but it is known that a family history of eating disorders, along with low self-esteem and characteristics of obsessive-compulsive disorder, may contribute.

Patients will appear extremely thin and may exercise excessively. Hair will be thin and nails will be brittle. The skin may be dry, and they may experience dizziness or syncope. Patients are often anemic and may have some electrolyte abnormalities. Menstruation may stop in females. Hypotension and cardiac dysrhythmias often develop.

Treatment is with psychotherapy to help patients develop a better self-image and learn healthy coping methods. Antidepressants may help with some of the symptoms. Close medical monitoring is necessary to detect any possible life-threatening effects of anorexia.

Bulimia nervosa

Bulimia nervosa is an eating disorder characterized by episodes of bingeing and purging. Patients will eat excessive amounts and then feel disgusted with themselves and induce vomiting. The purging may also be accomplished with abuse of laxatives or diuretics. It is not entirely clear what causes bulimia, but a family history of eating disorders, along with a low self-esteem and striving for perfection, can contribute.

Patients with bulimia may be thin or appear normal in size. Dental caries can occur because of damage from stomach acids during vomiting. Ulcers may develop in the throat and mouth. Electrolyte abnormalities can occur and may be life-threatening. Dehydration, hypotension, and cardiac dysrhythmias may also occur.

Treatment for bulimia is psychotherapy to develop an improved self-esteem and healthy coping methods. The only medication that is indicated for treatment of bulimia is Prozac®, though anti-anxiety medications may also be helpful. Close medical monitoring is necessary to detect any life-threatening effects of bulimia.

Adjustment mood disorder

An adjustment disorder is a stress and anxiety condition that occurs in response to some change in a person's life. Most people adapt to change with minimal stress-causing symptoms, but people with adjustment disorder develop excessive symptoms with minimal change in their lives. The cause of adjustment disorder is not known.

Adjustment disorder will cause patients to exhibit signs of anxiety and depression in response to change. Patients may complain of sleep disturbances, extreme sadness, anhedonia, irritability, or even thoughts of suicide. They may exhibit behavior changes that are erratic, such as abusing drugs or alcohol, avoiding family, getting into legal or financial trouble, or destroying property. Children with adjustment disorder may have failing grades or may skip school.

Treatment is with psychotherapy to help work through the stress caused by the change in their lives and to develop healthy coping skills. If symptoms are severe, antidepressants may be helpful in relieving the symptoms of depression.

Major depression

Depression is a common illness, and most patients experience more than one major depressive episode in a lifetime. Patients with major depression often have repeated episodes of depressive symptoms that are difficult to treat. The causes of major depression include a positive family history, imbalances in the neurotransmitters in the brain, and possibly environmental factors, such as tragedy in one's life.

Symptoms of depression include anhedonia, sleep disturbances, unintentional weight loss or gain, crying for no reason, vague somatic complaints, and loss of concentration. Patients with major depression may develop irritability, restlessness, impatience, extreme fatigue, or low self-esteem.

Treatment is with a combination of psychotherapy and antidepressant medications. In-patient treatment may be necessary in those contemplating suicide. Compliance with treatment is essential to prevent repeated episodes of the symptoms of major depression. It should be noted that suicide rates tend to be higher in patients as they are "coming out of" an episode of major depression, when their mood and outlook on life seem to be improving.

Dysthymic mood disorder

Dysthymic mood disorder is very similar to major depression in its presentation, but the symptoms are not as severe. The symptoms must be present for at least 2 years without relief of symptoms for longer than any 2-month period. The cause of dysthymic disorder is not clearly understood, but may be due to a positive family history, imbalances in the neurotransmitters in the brain, and environmental factors, such as a loss of a loved one.

Symptoms vary, but generally patients will complain of sleep disturbances, unintentional weight loss of gain with a change in appetite, and chronic fatigue. Patients may have a low self-esteem with feelings of hopelessness.

Treatment of dysthymic mood disorder is with psychotherapy to help patients work out the cause of the depressive symptoms and develop healthy coping methods. Antidepressant medications can also be helpful in relieving the symptoms though compliance with treatment is necessary to prevent a reoccurrence of symptoms.

Bipolar disorder

Bipolar disorder is characterized by mood swings that range from major depression to mania. The severity of the disorder varies among patients, but it usually greatly affects a person's life. The exact cause of bipolar disorder is unknown, but it is thought that a positive family history, imbalances in the neurotransmitters in the brain, and some environmental factors may play a role in its development.

The "low" points of bipolar disorder cause the classic symptoms of major depression with anhedonia, sleep disturbances, feelings of hopelessness, and possibly suicide. The "high" points occur during the manic phase. The characteristics of mania include restlessness, lack of sleep, aggressive behavior, pressured speech, inflated self-esteem, erratic behavior, and possibly legal or financial trouble. Patients can swing back and forth from these two states very quickly and frequently.

Medical treatment of bipolar disorder is with mood stabilizers and antidepressants. Anti-anxiety medications may also be helpful. Some patients have responded well to anticonvulsants and antipsychotics.

Personality disorders

Antisocial personality disorder

People with antisocial personality disorder often repeatedly break the law, lie, cheat, steal, or harm others. They are often poor parents and are frequently imprisoned for their actions. The condition is most often noticed during the teenage years and symptoms tend to decrease as a person ages. It is more common in men and often develops in those who suffer abuse or neglect as a child.

Symptoms include impulsiveness, repeated lying, stealing, aggression, and violence. Patients may be irritable, easily bored, or depressed. Oftentimes, these people appear to be very charming and fun to be around, but they will unexpectedly lash out at others or have very violent temper tantrums.

Antisocial personality disorder is very hard to treat. A combination of psychotherapy with antidepressants or antipsychotics may help to control the symptoms. If patients are at risk of harming themselves or others, hospitalization with in-patient treatment may be necessary. The symptoms will often begin to decrease as patients enter middle age.

Avoidant personality disorder

Avoidant personality disorder is a condition in which a person is very anxious or fearful of any social situations. They may be obsessive or exhibit odd behaviors that prevent them from functioning appropriately in social situations. There is no definite known cause, but social and biological factors may play a role in the development of avoidant personality disorder.

These patients are often very uncomfortable in social situations and may appear to be extremely shy. They are very concerned about what others think about them and do not respond well to criticism or rejection. Interpersonal relationships are often very short-lived or do not occur at all because of their inability to overcome these feelings.

Treatment of avoidant personality disorder is with a combination of psychotherapy and antidepressants or anti-anxiety medications. Antipsychotics may be necessary if patients are exhibiting any psychotic features with their disease. Therapy can be difficult, though, because of their difficulty with forming trusting relationships with therapists.

Borderline personality disorder

Borderline personality development is a condition in which a person struggles with maintaining an even personality. They are constantly in a conflicting state in which they cannot regulate their emotions. This condition is more prevalent in women and is thought to occur due to a combination of child abuse or neglect, a positive family history, or a serotonin imbalance in the brain.

Symptoms of borderline personality disorder include a rollercoaster of mood swings. They may be happy with their life situation one day and hate it the next day. This makes relationships very difficult. They frequently change jobs or move. They often have a low self-esteem and may even have tendencies to hurt themselves.

Treatment of borderline personality disorder is with a combination of psychotherapy and medications. Antidepressants and anti-anxiety medications can help control some of the symptoms. Hospitalization may be necessary if patients are at risk of harming themselves.

Histrionic personality disorder

Histrionic personality disorder is a condition in which a person is extremely emotional or dramatic. The condition is more common in women than men, and the cause is not completely understood though it is probably due to a combination of genetic and environmental factors.

Symptoms of histrionic personality disorder include an obsession with the approval of others. These patients often are very dramatic and attention seeking. They may wear very revealing clothing and act out in a sexually promiscuous way. They may have multiple sexual partners and not become emotionally attached to any one person. They can have frequent mood changes and be impulsive.

Treatment of histrionic personality disorder is often with a combination of psychotherapy and medications. Psychotherapy can be difficult because of patients' inability to form trusting relationships with the therapists. Antidepressants and anti-anxiety medications may help with the symptoms. Hospitalization may be necessary if patients are in danger of harming themselves.

Narcissistic personality disorder

Narcissistic personality disorder is a condition in which people have no regard for others and feel that they are superior to others. It occurs more frequently in males than females, and symptoms often become evident in early adulthood. Narcissistic personality disorder may be caused by abuse or neglect as a child or possibly from excessive pampering and spoiling as a child. It may also be related to an imbalance of neurotransmitters within the brain.

Symptoms of narcissistic personality disorder are a combination of extreme boastfulness and conceit but with a very volatile self-esteem. Criticism from others can be devastating, but these patients will often put down those who do not praise them. They belittle others and have difficulty maintaining healthy relationships. These patients often praise their own achievements and take advantage of others to get what they want.

The primary treatment for narcissistic personality disorder is psychotherapy. If there is underlying depression or anxiety, medications to treat these conditions may be helpful.

Paranoid personality disorder

Paranoid personality disorder is characterized by odd or eccentric behaviors that interfere with daily living. Risk factors include a positive family history of the disorder. Environmental factors, such as a history of child abuse or neglect, may also play a role in developing paranoid personality disorder.

Symptoms of paranoid personality disorder include distrust of others, extreme sensitivity to criticism, and irritability. These patients often feel that others are "out to get them" and may find criticism in even the most innocent remark. They have difficulty maintaining healthy relationships and do not work well with others. They often isolate themselves emotionally from others because of the perception that others are out to hurt them.

Treatment of paranoid personality disorder is with a combination of psychotherapy and medications. Antidepressants, anti-anxiety medications, and antipsychotics may be helpful in controlling some of the symptoms. Therapy can be difficult because of patients' inability to form trusting relationships with therapists.

Schizoid personality disorder

Schizoid personality disorder is a condition in which people withdraw from society and avoid interaction with others. They often find relationships too distressing and feel more comfortable when they are isolated. The cause is thought to be extreme child neglect or abuse. They may have had parents who were uninvolved in their lives and did not exhibit any love toward them.

Symptoms of schizoid personality disorder include self-imposed social isolation, a lack of social skills, indifference to criticism, and inability to maintain healthy relationships with others. They often have a flat affect and show very little emotion. These patients may have a low work ethic and be poor students.

Psychotherapy is the mainstay of treatment with schizoid personality disorder. This is focused on developing social skills and helping patients find pleasure from interacting with others. Medications may be used to help treat some of the concomitant symptoms of depression or anxiety.

Schizotypal personality disorder

Schizotypal personality disorder is a condition in which people isolates themselves from social situations because of extreme anxiety when interacting with others. They find their isolation very distressing, though, unlike the schizoid personalities who crave isolation. Risk factors include a combination of a family history of schizophrenia or environmental factors, such as abuse or neglect during childhood.

Symptoms of schizotypal personality disorder include social isolation, anxiety and distress with isolation or social interaction, and a lack of relationships with others. These patients often develop a belief that they have magical powers, such as mental telepathy, and may exhibit odd behaviors. Their emotions may be unstable with occasional temper tantrums or rages.

Treatment is with a combination of psychotherapy and medications. Antidepressants and antipsychotics may help to relieve some of the symptoms of this condition. Therapy can be difficult because of patients' inability to develop trusting relationships with therapists.

Obsessive-compulsive disorder

Obsessive-compulsive disorder (OCD) is a condition in which a person performs repeated activities or has obsessive thoughts that interfere with their daily lives. The condition frequently begins during adolescence and may be due to several factors. Environmental or genetic factors can increase the tendency to develop OCD. Low serotonin levels may also play a role. Excessive stress and disruption in one's life can lead to OCD. There is some preliminary research that shows there may be a link between *streptococcal* throat infection and the development of OCD.

Symptoms comprise obsessions and compulsions:

- Obsessions are thoughts that are constant, anxiety-provoking, and interfere with a person's ability to concentrate.

- Compulsions are the actions that come about because of the obsessive thoughts. These can be excessive washing and cleaning because of obsession with germs, or any other repetitive actions.

Treatment is psychotherapy and antidepressants. Both Paxil® and Zoloft ®have been approved for the treatment of OCD. These medications help to elevate serotonin levels in the brain.

Delusional disorder

Delusional disorder is a condition in which a person develops very strong beliefs in a specific situation that is not true, to the point that they alter their behaviors and life around this idea. This disorder may be caused by a combination of environmental or genetic factors though no specific cause is understood.

Delusional disorder can take different forms. Patients may have delusions of grandeur, believing that they are above everyone else and in a much higher standing than they really are. They may have paranoid delusions that others are out to hurt them or others. They may have a belief that someone is in love with them. They may also have delusions that they are physically ill when there is nothing medically wrong.

Treatment is with a combination of psychotherapy and medications. Antidepressants and antipsychotics may help to control the symptoms. Treatment can be difficult because patients firmly believe in their delusions.

Schizophrenia

There are 5 primary classifications of schizophrenia:

- Paranoid-type is characterized by delusions and auditory hallucinations. Functioning and affect are usually normal, but these patients may believe that they are at risk of being harmed by others or may have delusions of grandeur.
- Disorganized-type is characterized by inappropriate behaviors or expressions. They may laugh or cry at inappropriate times, and these actions can interfere with their daily lives.
- Catatonic-type is characterized by abnormal movements. These patients will remain still and not speak, or they may have repeated movements that do not make sense. They may also repeat the same words or phrases over and over (echolalia).
- Undifferentiated-type is characterized by combined symptoms of all the types of schizophrenia, but not consistently so as to label it as another type of schizophrenia.
- Residual-type occurs when patients have had at least one prior episode of schizophrenic behavior but is not currently having any symptoms. This can occur between episodes or may occur without any other future episodes of these behaviors.

Schizoaffective disorder

Schizoaffective disorder is a combination of schizophrenic symptoms with a mood disorder. These patients may have hallucinations and delusions with depression, anxiety, or mania. The condition is thought to be caused by a combination of genetic, environmental, and biologic factors.

Schizoaffective disorder will cause patients to have delusions and/or hallucinations consistent with schizophrenia. Along with these behaviors will be major depression, extreme anxiety, or episodes of mania. Patients may cycle between depression and mania, consistent with a bipolar component to the condition. Symptoms may become severe enough that patients can be at risk for harming themselves or others.

Treatment of schizoaffective disorder is with a combination of psychotherapy and medications to control the symptoms. Antidepressants, anti-anxiety medications, or antipsychotics may be used depending on patients' symptoms. Medications to stabilize mood may also be useful in decreasing the mood disorder component of the disease. Hospitalization may be necessary for in-patient treatment, especially if patients are at risk of hurting themselves or others.

Pulmonary

Acute bronchitis

Acute bronchitis is an infection of the bronchial tree. This infection and inflammation causes the bronchial structures to secrete more mucus, which causes wheezing and a productive cough. This infection is usually caused by a virus.

Patients with acute bronchitis will complain of a chronic cough, usually productive, and may describe some wheezing. They may have developed the common cold and feel that this has now started with symptoms in their lungs. They may say that the cough is worse at night and may or may not have a fever with this.

Because acute bronchitis is usually caused by a virus, antibiotics rarely help to relieve the symptoms. Using a humidifier at night to moisten the air, drinking plenty of fluids to thin the mucus secretions, and resting should help to relieve the symptoms within a week. The cough of bronchitis may linger for several weeks as the bronchial tubes heal.

Acute bronchiolitis

Acute bronchiolitis is a viral infection that causes inflammation of the upper and lower respiratory tract. This most often affects infants and young children because older children and adults have larger bronchial tubes that can accommodate this inflammation and the edema associated with it. Respiratory syncytial virus (RSV) is one of the viruses that can cause acute bronchiolitis in children.

The parents of patients with acute bronchiolitis may describe hearing their child wheeze and cough frequently. The child may even appear short of breath. A low-grade fever is usually present. Rarely, the severe respiratory symptoms can lead to respiratory arrest.

The cause of acute bronchiolitis is usually viral, so treatment is supportive with nebulizer treatments to decrease the inflammation and open the airways. Humidifier use to moisten the air can be helpful also. Antipyretics should be given to decrease fever, if present. Plenty of fluids should be given to prevent dehydration.

Acute epiglottitis

Acute epiglottitis is a medical emergency that can result in the epiglottis blocking the trachea if it is not treated immediately. It can be caused by the *H. influenzae* bacterium, but this is not often seen because of the immunization now available. *Streptococcus* and *Staphylococcus* are the most common bacteria to cause epiglottitis now. Trauma to the throat can also cause inflammation of the epiglottis.

Patients with epiglottitis will have a muffled voice. There will be throat pain and usually a fever. Difficulty swallowing and breathing will also be present. Patients lean forward to breathe and may even be drooling if swallowing is too difficult. If epiglottitis is suspected, one should NOT attempt to visualize the epiglottis because this may cause more inflammation and could close the airway. Lateral neck x-rays will show an enlarged epiglottis (thumb sign).

Treatment is with second and third-generation cephalosporins. Patients should be kept calm, should avoid swallowing or talking, and intubation equipment should be kept on hand in case of airway obstruction.

Pertussis

Pertussis, or whooping cough, is a highly contagious respiratory infection caused by the bacterium *Bordetella pertussis*. Pertussis is becoming more common now because immunization from the DPT injection tends to wear off by adulthood.
The symptoms come in 3 stages:

- The first stage, the catarrhal stage, is when there are symptoms of a cold such as runny nose, fever, sneezing, and mild cough.
- After one to two weeks, the second stage, or paroxysmal stage, begins. This is characterized by coughing spells that often leave the person breathless. These spells are followed by a loud inspiratory breath that makes a loud "whoop" sound.
- The third stage, or convalescent stage, lasts two to three weeks as the symptoms gradually fade. It is questionable whether antibiotics help to shorten the duration of symptoms of pertussis. Erythromycin can be given for 7 days to help eradicate the bacteria. There are no proven effective treatments to treat the cough.

Croup

Croup occurs because of inflammation around the larynx and trachea. It occurs in children and causes a cough that sounds like a bark and is very distinguishable. It is most often caused by the parainfluenza virus, though sometimes by RSV, measles, or bacterial infections. The barking cough associated with croup is usually worse at night and can wake a child up from sleep. A fever and hoarseness are usually present. If children are old enough, they will complain of sore throat.

Humidified air and cool drinks will help to ease the inflammation in the throat. Keeping children calm and decreasing the amount they talk will also help relieve the irritation. Sometimes, nebulizer treatments with corticosteroids or epinephrine can help to dilate the airways. Rarely, hospitalization is necessary with oxygen tent treatments or even intubation if very severe. In the rare case that bacteria is the cause of croup, appropriate antibiotics can be given to eradicate the causative organism.

Asthma

Asthma occurs when the airways are inflamed. These airways will constrict and produce more mucus, which causes difficulty breathing and the classic "asthma attacks." Asthma is frequently seen in multiple family members. It can be aggravated by allergen exposure, cold air, exercise, and stress.

The symptoms of asthma include wheezing, difficulty breathing, and chest tightness. Symptoms may be worse during the night. Coughing spasms can also occur as the airways constrict and the lungs attempt to expel the extra mucus that is produced.

Treatment can be divided amongst long-acting medicines and quick-acting "rescue" medications. The long-acting drugs used include inhaled corticosteroids, beta-2 agonists, leukotriene modifiers, and Cromolyn®. The short-acting medications are used when patients are having an acute exacerbation of the disease and include short-acting beta-2 agonists, ipratropium (Atrovent®), and corticosteroids. The best treatment is prevention by minimizing exposure to known allergens or triggers, using medications regularly, and not smoking.

Pneumothorax

Pneumothorax usually occurs due to an injury or chronic condition, and is described as air in the space around the lungs. It is classified as "primary", "secondary", "traumatic", or "tension".

- A primary pneumothorax usually occurs in young, tall males. This happens when a bleb ruptures on the lung, causing collapse of a portion of the lung. This does not occur because of chronic lung disease. If small, it can be monitored with chest x-rays. If large, hospitalization with a chest tube may be necessary.
- A secondary pneumothorax occurs with chronic lung disease, such as COPD or cystic fibrosis. It can be life-threatening and may require a chest tube for treatment.
- A traumatic pneumothorax occurs when there is trauma to the chest wall that results in air entering the chest cavity. This can result in a small pneumothorax that can be monitored or it may be large enough to require a chest tube.
- A tension pneumothorax occurs when air becomes trapped in the pleural space and cannot escape. This will result in a worsening pneumothorax that will eventually cause the structures in the pleural cavity to shift. It can be life-threatening and should be treated urgently with a chest tube.

Influenza

Influenza is a viral infection that affects the entire respiratory system from the nose to the lungs. There are 3 strains of influenza virus: A, B, and C. Types A and B is the ones seen most often and the ones that the annual flu shot is most effective against. Type C is not as common.

Though the symptoms can be very similar, the flu and the common cold differ in that the flu is very sudden in onset while a cold tends to come on slowly. A patient with the flu will have a high fever with chills and sweats, body aches, nasal congestion, dry cough, headache, and loss of appetite. Children may also have vomiting and diarrhea.

Antibiotic treatment is not effective. Supportive treatment with rest, fluids, analgesics, decongestants, and cough suppressants can be tried. Usually the flu just needs to run its course, but it can linger up to several weeks. It can be life-threatening to the very young, the elderly, and the immunocompromised.

Pneumonias

Some classifications of pneumonia include:

- Bacterial pneumonia, or community-acquired pneumonia, is most commonly caused by *Streptococcus pneumoniae*. The balance of the cases of pneumonia is divided amongst *H. Influenzae*, *Moraxella catarrhalis*, atypical pathogens such as *Legionella* and *Mycoplasma* species, *Staphylococcus aureus*, and gram-negative organisms.

- Viral pneumonia is commonly caused by influenza A or B viruses. RSV can also cause viral pneumonia, as can the herpes virus, parainfluenza, adenovirus, and varicella viruses. Herpes and varicella virus pneumonias are rare.
- Fungal pneumonia is usually caused by *Histoplasma capsulatum*, *Coccidioides immitis*, or *Blastomyces dermatitidis*. This usually only occurs in those patients who are severely immunocompromised. Patients with this type of pneumonia often do not know they are infected until they become very ill.
- HIV-related pneumonia is most often caused by *Pneumocystis jiroveci*, though the immunocompromised patient is susceptible to contracting any type of pneumonia. Fungal pneumonias are also prevalent among patients with HIV.

Symptoms and treatments

Patients will present with symptoms of fatigue, productive cough with purulent sputum, fevers with chills, and dyspnea. Patients may have wheezes and crackles, fever, and a lung consolidation present on chest x-ray. Treatment of bacterial pneumonia is with antibiotics. There is growing resistance to many antibiotics, but first line treatment is with cephalosporins, macrolides, fluoroquinolones, or tetracyclines.

Viral pneumonia causes a low-grade fever with a cough that is mildly productive. Muscle aches are common. Patients may be sick for several days before seeing a doctor. Treatment of viral pneumonia can be done with an anti-viral such as amantadine or rimantadine if started within 36 hours of the onset of symptoms. Otherwise, treatment is symptomatic.

Fungal pneumonias have similar symptoms, but can also spread to become systemic. Treatment is with anti-fungals, depending on the infective organism.

HIV-related pneumonias have symptoms according to the type of pneumonia that is present. Treatment depends upon the infective organism.

Tuberculosis

Tuberculosis (TB) is more prevalent in those who are homeless or who live in crowded conditions. TB is seen more often in those who are frequently exposed to the disease. Under developed countries also have a higher prevalence of TB.

The symptoms of active TB include night sweats, chronic cough with hemoptysis, fever, fatigue, and dyspnea. Loss of appetite, weight loss, and pleurisy are often common. A person can be exposed to TB and not contract the disease but will test positive on a PPD skin test. Prophylactic antibiotics can be given at that time to prevent the development of symptoms.

Treatment of TB involves multiple antibiotics. INH and rifampin are mainstays of treatment and should be continued for at least 6 months of treatment. Pyrazinamide and ethambutol are also usually given. Once diagnosed, patients with TB should be kept in isolation, and the local health department should be notified of an active case of TB in the community.

Bronchogenic carcinoma

Bronchogenic carcinoma is the most deadly cancer in the United States and accounts for approximately 25% of all cancer deaths in this country. Bronchogenic cancer is primarily seen as lung cancer. Smoking is the most common risk factor, with almost all cases of this type of cancer occurring in smokers. Small cell carcinoma has the worst prognosis and has usually metastasized by the time it is diagnosed.

Symptoms include progressively worsening cough with or without hemoptysis and dyspnea. Weight loss and fatigue may be present as the disease progresses. If metastasis is present, patients may experience bone pain, abdominal pain, or confusion, depending on the location of the metastasis. Some small cell tumors may serve as an ectopic source of hormone production, so symptoms that mimic an endocrine disorder maybe evident.

Often, once diagnosed, prognosis is very poor with this disease. Treatment may involve surgery to debulk a large tumor or a lobectomy. This may be followed with radiation and/or chemotherapy depending on the location of the cancer.

Carcinoid tumors

Carcinoid tumors occur in the neuroendocrine system and are most frequently found in the appendix or small intestine, though they may also be seen in the lung or pancreas. They are slow growing tumors and are frequently not diagnosed for several years.

Patients with carcinoid tumors may be asymptomatic. If the tumor is outside the appendix, it will likely secrete serotonin, and symptoms of carcinoid syndrome can be seen (flushing, diarrhea, weight loss, loss of appetite, wheezing).

Treatment of carcinoid tumors consists of surgical removal of the tumor. This may involve an appendectomy or small bowel resection. Chemotherapy may be given if the tumor has spread to other locations in the body. Radiation can also be given but is usually reserved for those carcinoid tumors that have spread to the bones to help relieve pain. Interferon injections may be given to help decrease the growth of the tumor, especially if it is affecting the liver.

Bronchiectasis

Bronchiectasis is a condition in which the bronchial tubes are dilated which prevents people from being able to clear mucus from their lungs. Bronchiectasis can occur in just one location of the lungs or may occur in several areas. It is most often due to inflammation or infection, such as with pneumonia. Chronic disease, such as cystic fibrosis, can cause bronchiectasis. Patients will have a productive cough of yellowish green sputum or even hemoptysis, and they may be short of breath. With chronic disease, recurrent pneumonia in the same location of the lungs may occur.

If the bronchiectasis is due to chronic disease, regular postural drainage should be done to encourage drainage of mucus from the lungs. However, aspiration of a foreign body can damage the bronchial tubes. Inhaled corticosteroids can help to dilate the airways, and avoiding allergens can help to prevent further constriction of the airways. If due to pneumonia, appropriate antibiotic therapy should be given. In severe cases, a lobectomy can remove the damaged section of the lung.

Chronic bronchitis

Chronic bronchitis occurs when the bronchial tubes are irritated and inflamed, causing them to secrete excess mucus. This, in turn, causes the airways to become plugged and prevents adequate flow of oxygen.

Smoking is the most common cause of chronic bronchitis. Occasionally chronic exposure to dust and other irritants can cause chronic bronchitis.

Diagnosis is made by symptoms of a productive cough for at least 3 months during a 2-year period, most often in a smoker. This is not accompanied by an acute illness or cold symptoms, and patients are afebrile. Patients may complain of shortness of breath and occasional chest pain with wheezing. They may be chronically fatigued and have a feeling of general malaise.

Treatment is symptomatic and may include bronchodilators to widen the airways. Patients may require supplemental oxygen at home if hypoxia is severe. Patients should quit smoking to help decrease irritation to the lungs.

Cystic fibrosis

Cystic fibrosis is an autosomal recessive genetic disorder. It causes excessive mucus production that leads to lung obstruction, deficient enzyme production that causes pancreatic dysfunction, and a less-than-competent immune system.

Cystic fibrosis is diagnosed in childhood, usually after a child has had multiple lung infections or is exhibiting weight loss and failure to thrive. Symptoms include recurrent lung infection with excessive congestion, bowel obstruction due to thickened feces, and poor nutrition because of decreased vitamin absorption.

There is no cure for cystic fibrosis. Life expectancy is usually into the 20s, but advances in treatment have extended this somewhat. Postural drainage can be performed regularly to promote drainage of lung secretions. Enzymes are taken orally to aid in digestion. Bronchodilators and chronic steroids are given to decrease irritation in the lungs and promote bronchodilation. In severe cases, lung transplantation can be performed though this still does not cure the disease.

Emphysema

Emphysema occurs when the alveoli lose their elasticity and do not completely empty of air with expiration. This causes hyperinflation of the lungs with difficulty drawing in the oxygen needed to take another breath. The most common cause of emphysema is smoking. A deficiency in alpha-1-antitrypsin protein can also lead to emphysema.

Patients will feel short of breath and easily fatigued. They will have a chronic, mild, usually non-productive cough. Over time, patients will develop the appearance of a barrel chest and clubbing in their fingernails.

Treatment of emphysema includes inhaled bronchodilators to decrease the cough, though they are not as effective as they are with asthma. Steroids can help to decrease inflammation in the lungs, though they are not extremely effective. Quitting smoking is the best treatment to help prevent progression of the disease. Patients may require supplemental oxygen at home. Rarely, surgery can be done to remove the damaged tissue.

Pleural effusion

A pleural effusion is an accumulation of fluid in the pleural space. This can result in excessive pressure applied to the lungs. It is frequently caused by infections, such as pneumonia, or chronic disease, as seen with CHF or lung cancer.

Patients will complain of a cough and shortness of breath. They may have pleuritic chest pain. Decreased breath sounds may be heard, and there will be dullness to percussion over the lung fields. The effusion is evident on chest x-ray and may be better-examined by CT imaging.

Diuretics may be used to decrease the effusion if is it due to CHF. A thoracentesis may be done to draw the fluid off the lungs and to diagnose whether it is infective in nature or if it contains malignant cells. If the fluid is infective in nature, it could result in the formation of an abscess around the lungs. If the fluid collection increases, a pneumothorax can occur due to the pressure applied to the outside of the lung.

Pulmonary embolism

A pulmonary embolism (PE) occurs when a thrombus travels to the lungs and causes obstruction of the airway. PE can be caused by a deep vein thrombosis that travels to the lungs, by any conditions that cause the blood to be hypercoagulable, or by cardiac dysrhythmia.

Patients with a PE will become suddenly short of breath and may complain of chest pain, shoulder pain, sweating, or cough. On exam, the blood pressure may be low and there may be decreased breath sounds throughout the lungs. Patients may become unconscious.

Oxygen is given first to help patients. Blood thinners will also be started, usually heparin first. Injectable Lovenox® or oral Coumadin® may be given later. Patients will need to stay on Coumadin® because of the risk of recurrent PE. Once a PE is confirmed, "clot buster" thrombolytic drugs may be given to break up the clot. Throughout all treatment, medications may need to be given that will help keep patients' blood pressure at a normal level.

Pulmonary hypertension

Pulmonary hypertension is a rise in pressure within the pulmonary artery carrying blood to the lungs. It can be caused by left-sided heart failure, especially as the ejection fraction decreases and the left ventricular function decreases. There are many medical conditions that can also cause pulmonary hypertension, such as cirrhosis, sickle cell disease, scleroderma, and congenital heart disease.

The symptoms of pulmonary hypertension include shortness of breath, which becomes progressively worse, and fatigue. Patients may also complain of a cough, sometimes with hemoptysis, and may even have syncopal episodes. Chest pain may also occur as the condition becomes advanced.

The treatment of pulmonary hypertension focuses on treating the underlying cause. Treatment includes diuretics, beta-blockers, and ACE inhibitors for heart failure. Digoxin or other medications to improve cardiac function may also be helpful. Calcium channel blockers, vasodilators, and anticoagulants may also be useful in treating pulmonary hypertension and in preventing complications from this condition.

Cor pulmonale

Cor pulmonale is right-sided heart failure. This can occur because of prolonged pulmonary hypertension or an increase in pressure within the right ventricle. Chronic lung disease, such as COPD or cystic fibrosis, can lead to cor pulmonale.

Patients may complain of increasing shortness of breath and fatigue. They may have chest pain that is exacerbated with activity and that is not entirely relieved with rest as the disease progresses. On exam, patients may have an increase in jugular venous distention, ascites, hepatomegaly, or lower extremity edema.

The focus of treatment with cor pulmonale is to treat the underlying cause. Calcium channel blockers are generally given, and patients may require anticoagulant therapy to prevent complications of the condition. Vasodilators can also be given as can medications that will help to optimize cardiac function. Oxygen may be given for patients to use at home in order to supply their bodies with extra oxygen in order to improve oxygenation of the blood.

Pulmonary fibrosis

Pulmonary fibrosis is a condition in which the alveoli become damaged and are replaced by fibrotic scar tissue. This results in a thickening of the alveolar tissue, preventing the transfer of oxygen. The cause of pulmonary fibrosis is uncertain, but it is thought there may be a genetic tendency for people to develop this disease. It is also thought that inhaled environmental agents, including cigarette smoke, may increase the likelihood of developing pulmonary fibrosis.

Patients may complain of shortness of breath, especially during activity. They may have a dry, hacking cough and fatigue. Patients may have a loss of appetite with significant weight loss. On exam, there may be decreased breath sounds and a decrease in oxygen saturation with pulse oximetry.

There is no curable treatment for pulmonary fibrosis. Supplemental oxygen can be given to help with shortness of breath. In severe cases, a single lung transplant may be performed.

Pneumoconiosis

Pneumoconiosis is an occupational lung disease that is due to inhaling particulate matter. It can be due to inhaling the dust from coal, asbestos, silica, beryllium, iron, and other materials. The specific type of pneumoconiosis will vary depending upon the material inhaled. For example, asbestos workers can develop asbestosis while those who work with silica develop silicosis.

Patients will complain of progressively worsening shortness of breath that is more pronounced during activities. They will also have a chronic cough that may be productive or nonproductive. On exam, there may be decreased breath sounds present. Chest x-ray may show consolidated areas where the inhaled dust has damaged the lung tissue.

There is no known treatment for the pneumoconiosis diseases. Supportive treatment with supplemental oxygen may be necessary. Patients should avoid any future contact with causative substances and if they smoke, they should quit in order preventing any further damage to the lung tissue or any additional exacerbation of the illness. In very severe cases, lung transplantation can be performed.

Sarcoidosis

Sarcoidosis is an inflammatory disease that starts in the lungs but may go on to affect every organ system in the body. It is usually self-limiting and will resolve within a few years, but in rare cases it may be fatal. The cause of sarcoidosis is not known, but it is thought it may be due to an immune response after exposure to a certain bacteria, virus, or toxin.

Symptoms of sarcoidosis vary depending on the organ system affected. With lung disease, patients may complain of shortness of breath with a chronic cough. A skin rash, aching joints, weight loss, fatigue, and red or watery eyes may also be present. Lab tests may reveal an elevation in ACE and calcium, but this is not definitive for diagnosis. Bronchoscopy can be performed for granuloma samples and confirmation of the diagnosis.

Treatment cannot cure the disease but may help to control some of the symptoms. High-dose anti-inflammatory drugs are given and steroid therapy is necessary for treatment of severe symptoms.

Acute respiratory distress syndrome

Acute respiratory distress syndrome (ARDS) occurs when there is inflammation and fluid accumulation within the lungs. ARDS can be caused by pneumonia, trauma, shock, aspiration, or chemical burns. The onset of this condition is usually 1-3 days following the triggering event. ARDS can be life-threatening, and patients are treated in the ICU.

Patients will have rapid respiratory decline to the point of respiratory arrest. Patients may become unconscious and multisystem organ failure can occur. Patients may also be hypotensive, and cardiogenic shock can set in. On exam, crackles may be heard in the lungs because of fluid accumulation. Cyanosis is frequently present.

Maintaining proper oxygenation is the mainstay of treatment. Patients are usually placed on ventilators until they can be weaned off and are able to breathe on their own. If a lung infection is present, appropriate antibiotics should be given. Diuretics may be given to decrease the fluid accumulation within the lungs.

Hyaline membrane disease

Hyaline membrane disease affects premature infants. It occurs when infants are born before the lungs are producing adequate amounts of surfactant. Surfactant helps to prevent the lungs from collapsing. As the airways collapse, infants will struggle more and more to breath until they become acidotic and multisystem organ failure begins. The most common symptom of this condition is respiratory distress in the premature infant. Surfactant is usually present after week 35 of gestation, and amniotic fluid can be tested for adequate production of the substance. The baby can become cyanotic and become more dyspneic. Respiratory arrest can occur after the baby becomes exhausted.

Treatment of this condition includes mechanical ventilation with positive pressure. Artificial surfactant can be given through the endotracheal tube. Babies may suffer permanent respiratory illness because of hyaline membrane disease, but others make a full recovery and suffer no consequences. The best treatment is maintaining a healthy pregnant to prevent premature birth.

Aspiration of a foreign body

Aspiration of a foreign body is commonly seen in children. It can occur in patients with swallowing difficulties as they aspirate food, liquids, or medications because of dysphagia. Frequently patients will have a persistent cough and the feeling the something is "stuck" in their throats. Wheezing or stridor may be heard, depending on the location of the blockage within the airway. If severe, the airway may be completely blocked, and this could cause patients to collapse and go into respiratory arrest. On exam, decreased breath sounds may be present on one side due to blockage of the main bronchus. Wheezing may also be heard in any portion of the lungs.

Treatment is focused on removing the object. In severe cases, the Heimlich maneuver should be given to forcefully expel the object from the airway. In emergency cases, an emergency tracheostomy may be performed to create a new airway below the level of the obstruction. In patients who are stable, bronchoscopy can be performed to physically remove the object.

Reproductive

Endometriosis

Endometriosis occurs when the tissue that makes up the uterine lining is also present outside the uterus. This can occur on the fallopian tubes, the ovaries, or outside of the uterus. It will thicken with hormonal changes that occur during the menstrual cycle and will shed, causing irritation to the surrounding structures. When severe, endometriosis can cause adhesions and severe pain. The cause of endometriosis is unknown.

The most common symptom is cramping pain, especially during menstruation. Bleeding can be excessively heavy. Infertility may occur as scar tissue and adhesions form. These may interfere with normal release of the mature egg from the ovary.

Oral contraceptives can help maintain hormone levels to prevent excessive symptoms from this condition. Medications to prevent the secretion of hormones by the ovaries can also help to decrease the symptoms. Laparoscopic surgery can be done to remove the tissue from the ovaries and fallopian tubes and decrease the symptoms and increase chances of pregnancy. As a last resort, hysterectomy may be performed.

Metritis

Metritis is an infection of the uterine lining that occurs following childbirth, usually due to retained fragments from childbirth. It can be life-threatening if not promptly treated and should be considered as a diagnosis in any woman who develops a fever after childbirth.

The first symptom will be a fever with chills and patients may complain of lower abdominal or pelvic pain. The uterus will be tender on palpation and the vaginal discharge present will have a foul odor. This can develop rapidly into peritonitis, pelvic abscess, and septic shock. This can cause coagulopathies with possible deep vein thrombosis or pulmonary embolism.

Treatment is with prompt administration of multiple IV antibiotics. Blood transfusion may be necessary if septic shock develops. The antibiotics should be continued for at least 48 hours after the fever resolves.

Manual exam should be performed to attempt to remove any retained placental fragments, and surgery may be necessary to irrigate the uterus or to do a hysterectomy if symptoms do not resolve.

Ovarian cysts

Ovarian cysts are relatively common and occur on the surface of the ovaries. Most do not produce symptoms, but some women can have significant symptoms from these cysts. Cysts can occur in the follicle when the egg does not release from the maturing follicle and continues to grow, leading to a cyst. These generally resolve without treatment. A corpus luteum cyst occurs after the egg ruptures, and the follicle becomes the corpus luteum. It seals itself off and begins to expand as fluid accumulates in it to form a cyst.

The follicular cysts generally do not cause symptoms. The corpus luteum cysts, however, can grow to be 4 cm wide and may cause significant abdominal pain. These can also rupture, which will cause sudden, severe abdominal pain and syncope. Oral contraceptives may prevent cyst formation with the menstrual cycle by regulating hormone secretion. If symptoms are persistent, surgery may be necessary to remove the cysts from the ovary. If a cyst ruptures, removal of the ovary may be necessary.

Cervicitis

Cervicitis is inflammation or infection of the cervix. This usually occurs due to sexually-transmitted diseases, such as chlamydia or gonorrhea. Chemical irritation from lubricants, spermicides, or douching may also cause cervicitis. Bacterial vaginitis may also cause a bacterial infection of the cervix.

Patients will complain of lower pelvic pain that is aggravated during sexual intercourse. They may have noticed an increase in vaginal discharge that is yellow or grayish in color with a foul odor. Frequent, burning urination may be present. The inflammation of the cervix may cause bleeding between menses. Fever may or may not be present depending on the severity of infection.

A Pap smear with *Gonorrhea* and *Chlamydia* cultures should be done for definitive diagnosis. Appropriate antibiotics should be started to prevent spreading of the infection, which could lead to pelvic inflammatory disease or a pelvic abscess. If the irritation is chemical in nature, patients should stop using the causative agent.

Incompetent cervix

An incompetent cervix refers to a cervix that will not remain completely closed during pregnancy, placing the baby at risk for premature birth. This can be due to past trauma to the cervix, such as from surgery or D&C. Previous deliveries that were traumatic to the cervix may lead to an incompetent cervix, as can genetic anomalies that cause a malformed cervix.

Unfortunately, an incompetent cervix is usually diagnosed after a second or third-trimester miscarriage occurs. The incompetent cervix can usually be detected on prenatal ultrasound or pelvic exam. Patients may or may not have some bleeding in the second or third trimester.

The cervix can be reinforced with a cerclage procedure, which involves placing purse string sutures in the cervix to draw it closed. This affectively sutures the cervix closed to prevent premature dilation. These sutures are usually removed in the last few weeks of pregnancy to prevent tearing of the cervix as it tries to dilate.

Cystocele

A cystocele occurs when the supportive connective tissues separating the bladder and vagina weaken, leading to a prolapse of the bladder into the superior end of the vagina. This can occur after childbirth or after lifting heavy objects for a period of time. A chronic cough can repeatedly strain these connective tissues, leading to a cystocele. Obese women are more likely to develop a cystocele.

Patients may be able to feel a mass in the vagina, and there may be a feeling of pressure in the lower abdomen or pelvis. Stress incontinence may be present, especially when patients are laughing or coughing. If urine is being retained in the bladder, patients may develop recurrent urinary tract infections.

A pessary can be inserted to provide extra support to these connective tissues and prevent the bladder from prolapsing into the vagina. If symptoms are very bothersome and not relieved with more conservative measures, surgery may be necessary to strengthen the support underneath the bladder.

Rectocele

A rectocele occurs when the supportive connective tissue separating the rectum and vagina weaken, leading to a prolapse of the rectal wall into the vagina. This is usually due to any type of trauma that weakens the supportive tissue in this area, such as childbirth or repeated heavy lifting. In some women, the decrease in estrogen that occurs after menopause may cause laxity of these connective tissues, leading to a rectocele.

Patients may or may not experience symptoms from a rectocele, depending on its severity. There may be a sensation of a mass present in the vagina. Patients may have chronic constipation or have the sensation that the rectum is not completely emptied following a bowel movement. Occasionally, patients may experience episodes of fecal incontinence.

A pessary can be inserted to support the vaginal wall and prevent the rectum from bulging into the vagina. If symptoms are very bothersome, surgery may be necessary to strengthen the connective tissue.

Vaginitis

Vaginitis is an inflammation of the vagina that is not necessarily due to an infection. Though infection from bacteria, viruses, or yeast can cause this inflammation, it can also be due to decreased estrogen levels following menopause, causing the vaginal walls to be drier and easily irritated.

The symptoms will depend upon the cause of the inflammation, but all types will usually cause vaginal itching or burning and pain with sexual intercourse. Bacterial infections cause a foul-smelling vaginal discharge that may be grayish in color. Fungal infections cause a white curd-like discharge. Vaginal trichomoniasis infection can cause a green-yellow vaginal discharge. Menopause-induced vaginitis will cause itching and irritation of the vagina and painful intercourse. There may be pain present during urination, as well.

Treatment will vary, depending on the cause of the inflammation. Appropriate antibiotics or antifungals may be necessary for infections. Estrogen cream can help with the vaginal dryness that occurs after menopause.

Fibrocystic breast disease

Fibrocystic breast disease is a condition in which women develop lumps in the breasts that come and go. There is no increased risk of breast cancer in patients who have this condition. It is thought that the fibrocystic masses felt in the breasts may be due to changing hormone levels during the menstrual cycle. Patients will complain of a breast mass that may change in size, especially during their menstrual cycles. These masses are usually painful and may radiate into the axillae. The breasts may feel full and heavy. Occasionally there will be a small amount of greenish-brown nipple discharge. Ultrasound exam will show cystic masses within the breasts.

There is no definitive cure for fibrocystic breast disease. Wearing a bra with extra support may help to provide some pain relief. It is thought that caffeine may worsen the condition, so limiting caffeine in the diet may help. Women should be encouraged to perform monthly self-breast exams one week after a period when cysts are at their smallest.

Mastitis

Mastitis is a condition in which bacteria enter the breast tissue through a milk duct or a fissure in the skin, caused by breastfeeding. Mastitis usually occurs within the first few weeks of breastfeeding, but may occur later on, also. Rarely, this condition occurs in women who are not breastfeeding.

Patients will complain of a painful area of the breast that is reddened and warm. They may feel very fatigued with a fever generally >101°F. A burning pain may be present constantly or only while breastfeeding. On exam, patients will appear generally ill. The area of the breast infected will be edematous and erythematous. The location of the infection may appear indurated.

Appropriate antibiotic therapy should be given to treat the infection, with attention to the safety of the antibiotic while breastfeeding. Patients should be encouraged to continue breastfeeding and apply warm compresses to the infected area.

Abruptio placenta

Abruptio placenta occurs when the placenta prematurely begins separating from the uterine wall. It is a medical emergency that can place the unborn child and mother at risk. Frequently, the cause of the placental abruption is unknown. However, it can occur following some type of trauma that occurs, such as a bad fall or car accident in which there is some degree of trauma to the mother.

Patients will have a sudden onset of abdominal or back pain with uterine contractions that are very close together, usually one after another. Vaginal bleeding will occur, and there may be pelvic tenderness to palpation on exam. If ultrasound determines that the placental abruption is very minor and the child is stable, the mother may be closely monitored on bed rest. If the symptoms should worsen, however, treatment is to deliver the baby as quickly as possible, usually via emergency C-section. If the baby is at term developmentally, a vaginal delivery may be attempted if the child's heart rate is stable.

Ectopic pregnancy

An ectopic pregnancy occurs when a fertilized egg fails to implant in the uterine lining. It most often will implant within the fallopian tube but can implant within the ovary, abdomen, or down low in the neck of the cervix. An ectopic pregnancy often occurs without any known cause, but scar tissue or a malformation of the tube can cause this to occur.

Patients may or may not know they are pregnant. They will complain of gradually worsening abdominal pain, usually one-sided, with vaginal bleeding. Rupture of the fallopian tube can occur as the ovum enlarges, and this will cause severe stabbing pain on the affected side. Syncope may occur if the tube ruptures.

Treatment is removal of the ovum. An injection of methotrexate can reduce the size of the ovum and cause dissolution of the cells, but this may require more than one injection. If rupture of the fallopian tube occurs, emergency surgery will be necessary to attempt to repair the tube or remove it.

Placenta previa

Placenta previa occurs when the placenta forms very close to the cervix, or even overlies the cervix. A female who has scarring of the inner uterus may develop this condition because of scar tissue preventing attachment of the placenta higher in the uterus. A malformed uterus can also cause placenta previa to develop. Females carrying multiple embryos at once can also develop this condition.

Bleeding is the most common symptom present in pregnant women with placenta previa. The amount and duration of bleeding late in pregnancy will depend upon how much of the cervix is covered by the placenta. There is a risk of massive bleeding and danger to the unborn child if the cervix begins to dilate, causing the placenta to tear prematurely.

Treatment depends upon the severity of symptoms. Patients should be on bed rest, possibly hospitalized if the condition is severe. If bleeding is persistent, the baby should be delivered via C-section as soon as possible, even if premature, to prevent further fetal distress.

Premature rupture of the membranes

Premature rupture of the membranes is a condition in which the amniotic sac ruptures before labor begins. This refers to situations in which the female is at least at 37 weeks gestation. This can occur early and is called preterm premature rupture of the membranes. Premature rupture of the membranes can occur because of infection of the amniotic membrane. Patients with poor diet and lack of prenatal care are also more at risk. Smokers and women who abuse alcohol or drugs during pregnancy may also be at increased risk. Patients will experience a trickle or a sudden gush of amniotic fluid from the vagina. This may be accompanied by vaginal bleeding. Contractions are not present.

Treatment is bed rest and imminent delivery of the baby. Vaginal delivery can be performed if the baby and mother are stable. Pitocin may be needed to start contractions if they have not started within 24 hours after rupture.

Task Areas

History Taking and Performing Physical Exams

Cholesteatoma

The patient with a history of ear infections who presents with foul ear drainage, pain in or behind the ear, dizziness, hearing loss, or partial loss of muscle control on the affected side should be evaluated for cholesteatoma. This abnormal growth in the middle ear can cause severe pain and hearing loss that, if treated, can often be corrected. Evaluation might include a hearing and balance test, and a computed tomography (*CT*) scan of the mastoid. If left untreated, cholesteatoma can lead to permanent hearing loss through bone deterioration, abscess, meningitis, and even death. Treatment initially focuses on resolving drainage and treating infection. Surgical removal may also be required.

Ganglion cyst

Also referred to as a bible cyst, a ganglion cyst is more common in women than men and most often located on the back of the wrist. It can also be found on the underside of the wrist, in the finger, knee, ankle, and toe joints. Manifestation can be gradual or rapid and is most often accompanied by pain that gets worse with joint use. The normal size is 1 to 3 cm, and it can appear as one large, immovable lump or a cluster. The lump may grow more prominent when the joint is engaged. Thick, clear fluid can be aspirated from the cyst. Ultrasound can also be useful in determining the makeup of the cyst.

Paronychia

Paronychia is the most common form of finger/toe nail infection. Infection often occurs after trauma to the area by moisture or physical or chemical damage. The nail bed becomes red, swollen, and painful to the touch. If left untreated, yellow-green pus will begin to collect and form an abscess. This infection can spread to the entire finger. This type of infection may or may not cause systemic fever or chills. If the infection reoccurs after treatment, suspect a fungal causative agent.

Celiac disease

Mild symptoms can include a sense of abdominal discomfort and an increase in flatulence. Increasing severity manifests with abdominal distention, bloating, diarrhea, steatorrhea, weight loss, fluid retention, anemia, osteoporosis, abnormal bleeding, nerve damage, infertility, muscle weakness and cramping, and bone fractures related to malabsorption. Stools are often liquid, greasy, light-colored, very foul smelling, and tend to float on top of the toilet water. Confirmation of celiac disease can be obtained through biopsy of the small intestine or testing for anti tissue transglutaminase antibody (anti-tTG) or endomysial antibody (EMA). Supporting data are obtained through complete blood count (CBC), chemistry panel, cholesterol and triglyceride, and thyroid and bone density tests.

Lyme disease

The patient often presents with a history of tick bite; note a history of outdoor activities even if a bite doesn't seem evident. The ELISA test for Lyme disease confirms antibody presence. During the first stage of onset, the lesion will show a clear center and reddened edges at the point of the bite within the first week. The patient may complain of itching, chills, fever, malaise, headache, faintness, muscle pain, and stiff neck. In stage two (weeks to months after the bite), the bacteria has begun to spread throughout the body, causing increased muscle weakness in the face, pain and swelling in large muscles or joints, and an irregular heart rate. Widespread infection indicates stage three (months to years after infection). The first line of treatment is doxycycline possibly in combination with rifampin for two to four weeks. Stages 2 and 3 Lyme disease are treated with intravenous (IV) ceftriaxone. Erythromycin is used in the presence of a penicillin allergy.

Acute cholecystitis

The acute cholecystitis patient often presents with upper-right-quadrant, postprandial pain described as sharp, aching, or cramping. This pain occurs at a distance of two to four hours after a meal, particularly after fatty or greasy meals. The patient may also complain of nausea with or without vomiting. Palpation will show a positive Murphy's sign (tenderness in the upper-right quadrant made worse by taking a deep breath). Fever and epigastric pain may also be present. Diagnosis confirmation is made with a nuclear hepatoiminodiacetic acid (HIDA) scan to locate a functional obstruction of the cystic duct. Treatment involves pain and fever relief, fluids, and preparation for surgery.

Diverticulitis

More than half of Americans older than age 60 will have some degree of diverticulitis. The patient with diverticulitis generally presents with loss of appetite, bloating, cramping, and lower-left-quadrant abdominal pain. The pain is not exacerbated by meals, but nausea and vomiting can be present. Confirm the presence of fresh blood in the stool, rebound tenderness, and fever. Lab work will show an elevated white blood cell count. A computed tomography (CT) scan with contrast can help with confirmation and the extent of disease by showing inflammation, perforation, diverticulosis, and fatty deposits within the colon.

Congestive heart failure

Key identifiers for many cardiovascular disorders are the presence of cyanosis (peripheral and central) and pallor. These, combined with shortness of breath related to position (supine) and exertion, fatigue, fluid retention and swelling, changes in heart rate, weight gain and wheezing, and/or productive cough (white or pink fluid), all suggest the presence of congestive heart failure (CHF). Treatment priorities include oxygenation and fluid reduction with diuretics. Other priorities, depending on individual patient needs, might include anxiety reduction and blood pressure reduction.

Pyelonephritis

Most cases of pyelonephritis occur in women with unresolved urinary tract infections (UTIs). Beginning symptoms mimic that of a UTI: urgency, frequency, and painful urination. As the infection spreads to the kidneys, back or flank pain, fever, malaise, nausea and vomiting, and mental disorientation (among the elderly) develop. Other symptoms might include hematuria and noticeable odor or discoloration of the urine. Physical examination exhibits kidney tenderness. Urinalysis shows increased white blood cells, bacteria, and possibly blood. Ultrasound or CT scan can be helpful in detecting abscesses, stones, or blockages aggravating the condition.

Trigeminal neuralgia

Trigeminal neuralgia creates extreme pain, often described as stabbing or electric-shock-like, along one side of the maxillary and mandibular (near the nose and mouth) first brachial branch. This pain is typically sporadic at first but may become constant. Triggers of the pain may include sound, touch, or stimulation of the area through brushing teeth, chewing, drinking, eating, or shaving. Often, no cause is found. Underlying causes are more likely to be determined in patients younger than 40, generally multiple sclerosis or a swollen blood vessel or tumor providing pressure on the trigeminal nerve. Testing often includes magnetic resonance imaging (MRI) and trigeminal reflex testing. Treatment might include antiseizure medications, muscle relaxants, or tricyclic antidepressants. More aggressive treatment entails cutting or destroying part of the trigeminal nerve, electrostimulation, microcompression, tumor removal, or microvascular decompression.

Fibrocystic disease

Fibrocystic disease can occur in women as young as 18, but it is most common in women 30 to 50 years of age, and it can effect up to 70% of women. Bilateral breast changes are described as lumpy, bumpy, ropelike, or an uneven texture of the breast tissue. This texture is often classified as nodular or glandular. Nipple discharge may also be present. Nodules are most noticeable in the upper outside area of the breast and can radiate to the underarm area. These changes are considered a normal deviation and not indicative of any actual disease. However, it is important to emphasize self-exams and mammograms because these textures can mask the development of abnormal lumps. Swelling, increased definition of the lumps, and tenderness can occur premenstrually. Symptoms and palpable changes tend to disappear after menopause.

Mitral stenosis murmur

The best way to detect a mitral stenosis murmur is to have the patient roll slightly onto their left side (left lateral decubitus position) and use the bell of the stethoscope over the apex. This allows you to easily detect a loud S1 followed by low-pitched rumbling sounds distinctive to mitral stenosis. These sounds can also be brought on during a stress test or exercise. Exertional dyspnea will also be present. Patches of pink-purple discoloration (mitral facies) in the cheek area may occasionally be present; a bounding jugular pulse may also be visualized. The exam should also assess for heart failure, atrial fibrillations, infection, and embolism.

Auscultating the cardiac valves

The S1 or "lub" sound is created by the mitral and tricuspid valves.
The S2 or "dub" sound is created by the aortic and pulmonary valves. Heart sounds are created by the blood flow through the valves, not the valves themselves. So the best auscultation will occur where those reverberated sound waves produce the greatest effect, not at the anatomical point of the heart valve itself.

Aortic valve: Right second intercostal space, right-upper sternal border

Pulmonary valve: Left second intercostal space, left-upper sternal border

Mitral valve: Left fifth intercostal space, medial to left midclavicular line

Tricuspid valve: Xiphisternal junction, lower-left sternal border

Mesenteric ischemia

There are three major arteries feeding the small and large intestines; when one or more develops restricted blood flow, mesenteric ischemia results. The stomach and liver may also be affected. This disease is more common in patients older than the age of 60; in smokers; and in those who have coronary artery disease, peripheral vascular disease, high blood pressure, and elevated cholesterol. Other conditions that may contribute to the development of mesenteric ischemia include chronic low blood pressure, congestive heart failure, aortic dissection, coagulation, and blood vessel disorders. Chronic symptoms often begin as vague complaints; acute problems occur suddenly. Symptoms include severe postprandial pain, bloody diarrhea, and in acute cases caused by a clot, vomiting may also be present.

Uterine fundal height

Fundal height is measured from the top of the pubic bone to the top of the uterus. It's a simple and noninvasive way to help judge the health and growth of the fetus. Variances can indicate a breech or transverse presentation; oligohydramnios, hydramnios, or polyhydramnios; multiple births; or engagement into the pelvis in preparation of birth. Measured in centimeters, fundal height should closely correspond to the number of weeks in the pregnancy. The top of the fundus should be palpable above the pubic symphysis at 12 to 15 weeks, at the level of the umbilicus by 20 to 22 weeks, and finally at the level of the xiphisternum by 36 to 38 weeks.

Patient sexual history

Be comfortable with your own sexuality, and maintain an objective, nonjudgmental attitude. Clearly specify the privacy of information that the patient can expect during and after the interview. Do not assume marital status or orientation. Ask open-ended questions, provide examples that illustrate an acceptance, and signify a "no-wrong-answer" attitude that gives the patient permission to speak freely. Use terms that the patient understands, and be clear in your use of terms. Clarify any terms the patient uses that might be ambiguous.

Anorexia nervosa

Weight loss that continues even as the patient continues to express intense fear of gaining weight or being overweight, even if he or she is already underweight. The patient may have a history of an anxiety disorder as a child, an extreme need for perfection, or an absorption in exercise. Note poor memory or judgment, emaciation, dysmenorrhea, orthostatic hypotension, bradycardia, hypothermia, dry skin, and thinning or brittle hair and nails. Lab results can show decreased white blood count, hypochloremia, hypokalemia, increased blood urea nitrogen (BUN), and metabolic acidosis.

Conditions associated with heavy alcohol use

Health effects of alcoholism include:

- Anemia and malnutrition.

- Cancer. Scientists believe that the increased cancer risk is related to the conversion of alcohol into acetaldehyde, a potent carcinogen, in the body. This risk is also increased by smoking. The most common types include, mouth, throat, larynx, esophagus, liver, breast, and colorectal.
- Cardiovascular disease, high blood pressure, and abnormal clotting that increase the risk of myocardial infarction or stroke. Atrial flutter can occur with excessive use or withdrawal symptoms.
- Cirrhosis and pancreatitis.
- Dementia and other forms of impaired thinking.
- Depression.
- Seizures, even in the absence of epilepsy. Alcohol can also alter the effectiveness of seizure medications.
- Aggravated gout.
- Suppressed immune system and nerve damage.

Comprehensive cardiac/vascular patient assessment

1. Patient history: The best source of information about the history of his condition is the patient himself. Other resources might include past medical records and involved family members.
2. Physical exam: Execute a full, head-to-toe and symmetrical exam including inspection, palpation, percussion, and auscultation methods as appropriate.
3. Laboratory results: Typical laboratory tests include cardiac enzymes, clotting function, cholesterol levels, and therapeutic medication levels.
4. Diagnostic tests: Diagnostic tests can include x ray, computed tomography (CT) scan, magnetic resonance imaging (MRI), electrocardiogram (ECG), echocardiography (ECHO), myocardial perfusion imaging, and cardiac catheterization.

Qualities of pain

1. Quality: Have the patient describe the quality of the pain using words such as dull, stabbing, sharp, aching, throbbing, and burning.
2. Severity: Pain can be rated on a scale of 1 to 10 or by another assessment tool.
3. Location: Where on the body is the pain located, and does it radiate or shift?
4. Timing: When did the pain begin; is it constant, or does it come and go with a predictable or random frequency?
5. Causative factors: Is the patient able to pinpoint a precipitating event prior to the onset of pain?
6. Aggravating factors: Does the quality or severity of pain change with activity, position, stress level, or other varying conditions?
7. Alleviating factors: What effects do medications, position, or other noninvasive treatment interventions have on the amount of pain?
8. Related symptoms: Is the pain accompanied with nausea, dizziness, shortness of breath, or other closely related symptoms?

In-depth personal history

The following lists methods of questioning that encourage the patient to give an accurate, in-depth personal history:

- Open discussion: Promotes patient comfort by encouraging questions and feedback during the interview.

- Ask leading questions: Ask questions that require more than a "yes" or "no" answer, and give clear permission for the patient to speak freely about their health.
- Restate and summarize provided information in another way: Allows you to verify that your understanding of the given information is correct.
- Focus: Assisting the patient to concentrate on identifying his highest healthcare needs or make connections between healthcare behavior and larger priorities.
- Order and sequence: Verify cause and effect and timing of the events given in a patient history.
- Encourage self-evaluation: Allow patients to draw their own conclusions regarding information, and do not judge or try to educate at this point.
- Make observations: Providing commentary on the patient's physical, mental, and emotional demeanor to help them focus and give permission to discuss further aspects of their health or immediate needs.

Breast cancer

When assessing for signs indicating breast cancer, the practitioner should feel for a painless mass in the breast or surrounding tissue. The most common locations are directly beneath the nipple and the outer-axillary portion of the breast. Other indications can include changes in the appearance or texture of the breast and nipple. There may be an obvious lack of symmetry between breasts. Nipple areas can change color, texture, and orientation as well as produce discharge. Breast cancer most commonly metastasizes to the bone, liver, brain, and lung. Breast cancer patients face issues associated with body changes – loss of femininity and loss of sexual appeal and function.

Prostate cancer

The most common symptoms noted by the patient with prostate cancer are difficulty urinating and sexual dysfunction. Urination difficulties can include difficulty starting or stopping the flow of urine, decreased force of urine stream, or dribbling. With a loss of sexual function, many men also experience a perceived loss of masculinity. Blood may be detected in both urine and semen, and the patient may experience weight loss and painful bowel movements. Bone pain in the lower back or pelvis indicates metastasis.

Rectal exam reveals a palpable prostate that is enlarged, hardened, with a lumpy or uneven surface. Prostate-specific antigen (PSA) blood levels will also be elevated.

Tuberculosis

Tuberculosis is common among immune-suppressed patients. Physical symptoms include night sweats, unexplained weight loss, and fatigue. Pulmonary tuberculosis also shows a chronic cough with active sputum production. If left untreated, tuberculosis may also spread to other organs and cause neurological diseases such as meningitis, bone infections, and urinary bleeding. A positive tuberculin skin test signifies a previous exposure to tuberculin organisms. However, it cannot pinpoint a recent change from a negative status unless the positive test is a follow-up to previous negative test results. The skin test alone cannot accurately pinpoint the time of exposure. An initial tuberculosis diagnosis to identify the presence of an active disease state can be obtained by finding acid-fast bacilli in stained smear samples from sputum or other body fluids. The initial diagnosis is confirmed by isolating *Mycobacterium tuberculosis* on culture or rapid nucleic acid test probes.

Pain assessment and management

All patients have the right to appropriate assessment and management of pain. Caregivers should encourage all patients to report their pain and follow through with pain-relieving treatments. Assessments for pain must be appropriate for the individual patient and address all aspects of their pain. Both the patient and family should be included in the assessment process. The most accurate indicator of pain is the patient's own description. It is always subjective: The clinician should accept and respect the patient's report of pain. Each person's pain experience is unique and dependent on many contributing factors such as heredity, energy level, coping skills, and prior experiences. Physiological and behavioral observations should not replace information obtained directly from the patient when it can be communicated. Pain can be present without physiological evidence or cause; pain in such cases should not be immediately assigned to psychological causes. Chronic pain can create an overall lower threshold of tolerance for pain and other stimuli. Unrelieved pain has adverse effects on all aspects of the patient's life.

Physical examination

Inspection: Visual inspection with the naked eye and specialized equipment such as an ophthalmoscope to view physical features such as height, body mass, skin condition and color, breath frequency and quality, hair distribution, balance, gait, and presence of tremors or physical injuries.

Palpation: Examination by touch for pulses, organ size and location, pain response, temperature, and distinguishable masses.

Percussion: Further touch intervention using the fingers to create sound.

Auscultation: Auditory assessment with and without the assistance of a stethoscope generally focusing on cardiac, respiratory, and digestive systems. Other useful tools might include the use of Doppler to locate pulses that were difficult to palpate.
This general procedure varies slightly during assessment of the abdomen, placing auscultation before palpation and percussion. Other systems may not require the use of all four examination elements.

Obsessive-compulsive disorder

Obsessive-compulsive disorder (OCD), also known as obsessive-compulsive anxiety disorder, is defined as a series of unreasonable thoughts that lead the patient to execute repetitive behaviors. Whether or not the patient believes these actions will alter the imagined fears, they are unable to ignore or stop the action. Completing the compulsion allows them to lower their anxiety and stress levels.

OCD may occur when there is a family history of the disorder or as a result of stressful life changes. Test results may show decreased serotonin levels, increased activity in the frontal lobe (thought to trigger the obsessions), and increased caudate nucleus activity (responsible for the resulting compulsions).

Disorders associated with smoking

The diseases most commonly associated with smoking are lung cancer and chronic obstructive pulmonary disorder (COPD). Tobacco use is also responsible for an increased risk of mouth, throat, bladder, kidney, liver, stomach, and pancreatic cancers. It decreases blood flow by damaging both peripheral and cerebrovascular vessels, increasing the risk of heart disease, myocardial infarction, and stroke. Respiratory conditions include chronic bronchitis, emphysema, pneumonia, exacerbation of asthma, as well as respiratory infections and colds. It can also cause infertility, miscarriage, stillbirth, premature and low-birth-weight infants, as well as impotence in men.

Macular degeneration

Macular degenration, also referred to as age-related macular degeneration (AMD), is the leading cause of vision loss in the patient older than 55 years of age. Risk factors that increase the likelihood of a patient developing AMD include smoking, Caucasian descent, high blood pressure, increased cholesterol levels, and genetics. The macula, the most sensitive part of the retina, which provides sharp, central vision, is destroyed. Progression is often very slow and therefore goes undetected for an extended period. If the progression is faster, it is more likely to affect the vision in both eyes. Central vision and the ability to focus on fine detail are lost. This makes it difficult for the patient to drive, recognize facial features, read, or do other close-up work.

Disorders associated with obesity

A patient who is more than 20% over the highest weight allowance for his or her height is considered obese. In other terms, an adult is considered overweight when their body mass index (BMI) is between 25 and 29.9. Obesity is defined as a body mass index (BMI) of more than 30.

These patients are more at risk for heart disease; high blood pressure; stroke; diabetes; colon, breast, uterine, kidney and esophageal cancer; gallstones; osteoarthritis; gout; polycystic ovary syndrome (PCOS); sleep apnea; and asthma than the patient within normal weight parameters. These conditions often coexist. Metabolic syndrome describes the patient with a grouping of obesity, hypertension, and elevated lipids and blood sugar.

Endometriosis

Endometriosis occurs when the endometrial cells that make up the lining of the uterus begin to invade and grow in areas outside of the uterus. The tissue often implants itself on the ovaries, bowel, rectum, bladder, and the lining of the pelvis. Normal endometrial cells respond to the hormone changes by being sloughed off during the woman's period. Cells that have migrated may bleed, but they are not released from the body. They continue to grow with each new menstrual cycle. Pain is the presenting factor for this disease and can be present during the patient's period and for up to two weeks prior to the period. Pain may also be present during sexual intercourse or bowel movements. It may also present as back pain that appears unrelated to hormonal changes. The patient with endometriosis is likely to have begun menstruation at a young age, is nulliparous, and has frequent, prolonged periods.

Cushing's syndrome

Cushing's syndrome is a hormonal disorder resulting from the body's tissues being exposed to excessive amounts of cortisol, either naturally or from overproduction, or more often, prolonged steroid treatment. The result is increased body fat on the face, neck, and between the shoulder blades with disproportionately skinny legs and arms. Skin and bones become fragile with poor healing and increased pain with routine daily activities. Patients complain of fatigue, muscle weakness, increased thirst, increased urination, and mood changes. They present with elevated blood pressure and high blood glucose levels. Women may experience abnormal hair growth on the face, neck, chest, stomach, and thighs as well as dysmenorrhea. Men may experience erectile dysfunction and decreased fertility.

Many of these symptoms can be found in other conditions, so these patients should also be screened for diabetes, polycystic ovary syndrome, and metabolic syndrome.

Using Laboratory and Diagnostic Studies

Coarctation of the aorta

Magnetic resonance angiography is preferable in the older patient. Echocardiography is not conclusive, but it can be used to help measure peak pressure gradients. Computed tomography (CT) angiography is an option in postoperative patients with stents and surgical clips. It can also be ordered to identify associated lower extremity damage. X-ray identifies related cardiomegaly, pulmonary edema, and congestive heart failure (CHF). Laboratory workups might include cultures, urinalysis, electrolytes, blood urea nitrogen (BUN), creatinine, glucose, arterial blood gases, and serum lactate.

Aortic dissection

Aortic dissection is most common in individuals with uncontrolled hypertension complaining of sudden, intense, stabbing back pain. A difference in blood pressure between the extremities may also be noted. These symptoms should be treated as an emergency situation until aortic dissection is confirmed or ruled out by a computed tomography (CT) scan with contrast. Magnetic resonance angiogram (MRA) and transesophageal echocardiogram (TEE) may also be considered in order to obtain the clearest picture of the heart and surrounding vessels.

KOH preparation

Any patient presenting with a scaly rash should undergo a KOH test. A KOH (potassium hydroxide) preparation is an inexpensive and noninvasive test used to detect the presence of fungal infections on skin, hair, nails, and vaginal discharge. A minute scraping from the infected area is placed on a microscope slide with KOH and the solvent dimethyl sulfoxide (DMSO). Skin cells will be quickly dissolved, leaving behind only fungal cells that appear as thin branching structures (septate hyphae).

Hydrogen breath test

Excess hydrogen is produced when there is an overabundance of undigested sugars and carbohydrates present in the small intestine. This hydrogen passes through the small intestines into the main blood supply and then to the lungs to be excreted during exhalation. This excess amount can be measured as a convenient and reliable method to diagnose lactase deficiency, lactose intolerance, bacterial overgrowth in the small intestine, or abnormal rate of digestion. The patient is asked to fast for 12 hours prior to the testing. An initial breath sample is taken by having the patient blow into a balloon. A small amount of sugar is then administered, and the hydrogen levels on the breath are then measured at intervals of 15 minutes for up to 5 hours. Any increase in hydrogen production means that there is a problem with the sugar digestion. An extremely rapid increase may indicate food is traveling through the small intestines too quickly; two separate spikes in hydrogen production may indicate a bacterial infection of the small intestines.

Pertussis

Testing procedures differ between private clinical and public health settings. For the private clinic, the goal is to rapidly diagnose and treat any patient who may be at risk (PCR). At a public health level, more discrimination against false negatives is required (culture). The polymerase chain reaction (PCR) is a rapid method of diagnosis that detects the presence of the DNA sequences particular to *Bordetella pertussis* bacteria without requiring the presence of live bacteria. Inaccurate results are still possible however. Best results are obtained within the first three weeks of signs and symptoms (cough) appearing and must be performed before antibiotic treatment begins. Swabs or aspiration of mucus is obtained from the nasal passage. Cultures should be started immediately after collection, and all mucus should be disposed of properly within 24 hours of collection.

Hypothyroidism

The older woman presenting with fatigue, dry skin, constipation, and/or a hoarse voice should be screened for hypothyroidism. Thyroid stimulating hormone (TSH) is the most sensitive test. A high TSH result (4.0 and above) is indicative of a thyroid with reduced function. Other laboratory workups might include triiodothyronine, thyroxine, triiodothyronine uptake, thyroxine-binding globulin, and anti-thyroid peroxidase (anti-TPO). Ultrasound of the thyroid may also be considered. Infertility, pregnancy, and mental and cardiac health also require a higher level of monitoring.

Cystic fibrosis

Cystic fibrosis is an autosomal recessive disease with mutation of chromosome 7. This particular chromosome is responsible for the transport of chloride across membranes. Failure to move chloride appropriately results in increased lung secretions and eventual fibroid and cyst formation. The immunoreactive trypsinogen (IRT) blood test is a standard screening procedure for newborns. High IRT test results warrant further testing through the sweat chloride test, the industry standard diagnostic test. X-ray and CT scan show tubular, air-filled pockets, normally in the upper lobes of the lungs. Lung, pancreas, and intestinal function tests, and a fecal fat test may also be ordered and monitored.

First-degree heart block

A first-degree heart block is generally asymptomatic, and it is often found in young, athletic individuals or those with increased vagal tone. Other causes for first-degree heart block include: avascular necrosis (AVN) disease, infection, myocardial infarction (often of the inferior wall), myocarditis, electrolyte imbalances, or medication (particularly antiarrhythmics). First-degree heart block is defined by an increased PR interval greater than 0.21 seconds with all atrial impulses conducted. Every beat is conducted, and there are no dropped beats, but the rate of conduction is slower than normal rates. If the PR interval is greater than 0.3 seconds, the patient may experience exertion, or exercise, intolerance. Upon physical exam, a slightly dampened S1 and/or diastolic murmur may be present.

Paroxysmal supraventricular tachycardia (PSVT)

PSVT refers to occasional, intermittent rapid heart rate that lasts from a few minutes to several hours. This most often occurs in younger patients, or can be brought on by alcohol, caffeine, smoking, illicit drug use, or digitalis toxicity. This condition does not necessarily indicate heart disease. Intervention of any kind might not be needed unless the patient is presenting symptoms such as anxiety, dizziness, shortness of breath, an uncomfortable feeling of chest tightness or racing heart, or fainting. Emergency treatment options might include the Valsalva maneuver (instructing the patient to attempt to forcibly exhale while keeping the mouth and nose closed), splashing the face with ice water, intravenous adenosine, or cardioversion. Long-term stability may be maintained by oral medications such as propafenone, flecainide, moricizine, sotalol, and amiodarone, the use of a pacemaker, or more often, radiofrequency catheter ablation.

Spirometry

Spirometry is an inexpensive and rapid way of assessing the extent and severity of airway obstruction causing a patient with asthma, chronic obstructive pulmonary disease (COPD), bronchitis, emphysema, or pulmonary fibrosis to be unable to expire as forcefully or as quickly as a normal person. These measurements are taken at the time of initial diagnosis and are then monitored periodically to track disease progression. Decreased forced expiratory volume (FEV-1), a measure of the amount of air expelled in a single second, decreased forced vital capacity (FVC), a measure of the largest amount of air you are able to expel, and a decreased FEV1:FVC ratio all indicate the severity of the breathing restriction. Measurements may be also reevaluated 15 minutes after administration of an inhaled bronchodilator to assess its specific effectiveness.

Holter monitor

A Holter monitor is worn continuously for 24 to 48 hours. This is helpful when a regular, brief electrocardiogram (ECG) has not shown any abnormalities, but the patient is presenting with symptoms such as pain, dizziness, palpitations, or a change of consciousness that could still be cardiac health related. While it does allow for an extended view and perspective on heart health, it is also partially dependent on accurate reporting/journaling on the part of the patient while wearing the monitor. It may also be a little bothersome to the patient, and he or she will not be able to shower or bath until the monitor is removed at the end of testing.

Atrial arrhythmias

Atrial arrhythmias are the most common type of cardiac arrhythmia. These include Premature atrial contractions (PACs): Normal rhythm, irregular rate with irregular P waves. The patient may complain of a "fluttering" sensation or exhibit low blood pressure.

Atrial flutter: A form of supraventricular tachycardia. Atrial rate of 250 to 400 beats per minute. Saw-toothed appearance on ECG. The critical nature increases with higher ventricular rates. The pulse may be normal, but the patient exhibits signs of decreased cardiac output.

Atrial fibrillation (A-fib): Chaotic electrical impulses of the atrium with a rate of 400 to 600 beats per minute and irregular ventricle rate. Cannot identify or measure P wave, PR interval, T wave, or QT interval. There is a high risk for shock, heart failure, or embolism. Pulses may not match the audible heart rate. The patient exhibits low blood pressure and change of consciousness.

Atrial tachycardia: A form of supraventricular tachycardia. Exhibits a regular atrial and ventricular rate between 150 to 250 beats per minute. Patient shows decreased cardiac output and is at risk for angina, heart failure, or myocardial infarction. A common cause is digoxin toxicity.

Sinus node arrhythmias

As seen on electrocardiogram (ECG)
The sinus node is the primary pacemaker for the heart, setting a normal rate and rhythm between 60 to 100.

Sinus arrhythmia: The electrocardiogram (ECG) rate falls within normal limits, but there is a slight change in rhythm correlating to breathing (increased pulse with inspiration, slowing with expiration).

Sinus bradycardia: The rhythm is normal, and all parts of the ECG appear normal with a rate below 60 beats per minute.

Sinus tachycardia: Rhythm is normal, ECG is normal, but the rate is greater than 100 beats per minute.

Sinus arrest: The rate is normal, but the rhythm is interrupted by occasional missing PQRST complexes. This is referred to as a sinus pause if only one or two beats are dropped; sinus arrest refers to three or more missing complexes.

Sick sinus syndrome: Irregular rhythm in which the waves and complexes vary instead of forming a predictable pattern.

Junctional arrhythmias

As seen on electrocardiogram (ECG)
Premature junctional contraction (PJC): The rate and rhythm are fundamentally regular with occasional early, inverted P wave and following QRS complex.

Junctional escape rhythm: Regular rate and rhythm appears to be normal sinus rhythm except for inverted P waves.

Accelerated junctional rhythm: Regular rhythm of 60 to 100 beats per minute. P wave may be absent or appear inverted before or after the QRS complex. Everything else appears normal.

Junctional tachycardia: Regular rhythm with a rate between 100 and 200 beats per minute. The P wave is inverted and occurs after the QRS complex.

Ventricular arrhythmias

As seen on electrocardiogram (ECG)
Premature ventricular contraction (PVC): Underlying regular rate and rhythm, with occasional early, wide, and bizarre looking QRS complex.

Ventricular tachycardia: No P wave, wide and bizarre QRS complex with rapid rate of 100 to 200 beats per minute.

Ventricular fibrillation: No identifiable rhythm, no identifiable waveforms. The electrocardiogram (ECG) shows only a fine or coarse chaotic wavy line. The patient is unresponsive and pulseless.
Idioventricular rhythms: Ventricular rate between 20 and 40 beats per minute, independent or no P wave (PR interval is unmeasurable) with a bizarre-looking QRS complex longer than 0.12 seconds.

Asystole: No electrical conduction displayed as an almost flat line only disturbed by medical interventions such as cardiopulmonary resuscitation (CPR). The patient is unconscious and pulseless.

Heart blocks

As seen on electrocardiogram (ECG)
First-degree AV block: The rhythm is regular and appears very similar to a normal sinus rhythm. The only difference is a PR interval longer than 0.20 seconds.

Type I second-degree AV block: Regular atrial rhythm with a repeating pattern of progressively longer PR intervals until a QRS complex no longer appears behind the P wave.

Type II second-degree AV block: Atrial rhythm is regular, ventricular rhythm may be either regular or irregular. Look for missing QRS complexes.

Third-degree AV block: Atrial and ventricular rates are regular, but they are independent of each other. The PR interval will vary.
Left bundle-branch block: The QRS complex is wider than 0.12 seconds; the R wave may not be detected or "slurred." Right bundle-branch block: The QRS complex is wider than 0.12 seconds and has an unusual appearance (may look like rabbit ears or the letter M). The T wave is inverted.

***Clostridium difficile* infection**

Clostridium difficile (*C. diff*) is a gram-positive, anaerobic, spore-forming bacillus that causes diarrhea and colitis. The proliferation of *C. diff* is usually the result of antibiotic therapy and is seen most often in the elderly patient. There can be an extended period of time (weeks to even months) before the patient even shows signs and symptoms of the infection. The bacteria release toxins that increase mucosal inflammation and damage to the colon. The patient presents with frequent diarrhea, and abdominal discomfort. In advanced cases, fever, nausea, dehydration, weight loss, and blood or pus in the stool will also be present. If symptoms are severe or persistent, they may need to be treated with metronidazole (first choice) or vancomycin.

Rheumatic heart disease

Rheumatic heart disease, caused by a streptococcal infection (generally in children), most frequently affects the mitral valve causing stenosis and regurgitation. Stenosis is created by inflammation of the valve leaflets, fibrin deposits on the cusps, fusion of leaflet adhesions (commissures) and formation of the classic "fish-mouth deformity" to the valve. X ray, computed tomography (CT), and magnetic resonance imaging (MRI) will show edema or inflammation in the acute phase, calcifications, cardiomegaly, specific chamber enlargements in established disease, and in severe cases pericardial effusion and alveolar hemorrhage.

CT scan

A computed tomography (CT) scan is a more detailed and intricate series of x-rays that allow for examination of bones and soft tissues. While there are often more cost-effective screening methods, CT scan is the first choice in the presence of a head injury. Other uses might include diagnosing muscle and bone disorders, internal injuries, and bleeding. It can also detect and monitor tumors, infection, blood clots, and heart and lung disease. A CT scan is not recommended in the pregnant patient. CT creates radiation exposure and creates a risk of an allergic reaction to any contrast used.

Electrocardiogram technique

Electrocardiography, or the electrocardiogram (ECG), is the study of electrical impulses through the heart. Correct placement of the 12 monitor leads must be executed in order to receive accurate results. Leads are divided into three divisions:
Limb leads—leads I, II, and III.
Augmented leads—aVR, aVL, and aVF.
Precordial leads—V1 to V6.

- V1 is placed at the fourth intercostal space, to the right of the sternum.
- V2 is also in the fourth intercostal space, to the left of the sternum.
- V3 is located directly between V2 and V4.
- V4 is placed in the fifth intercostal space at the midclavicular line.
- V5 is also in the fifth intercostal space at the anterior axillary line directly between V4 and V6.
- V6 is also in the fifth intercostal space at the midaxillary line.
- Additional leads are placed on each limb.

Normal ranges of a complete blood count (CBC)

White blood cells (WBCs):

- 4500 to 11,000/mm^3

Red blood cells (RBCs):

- male, 4.3 to 5.9 million/ mm^3
- female, 3.5 to 5.5 million/ mm^3

Hemoglobin (HGB):

- male, 13.5 to 17.5 g/dL
- female, 12.0 to 16.0 g/dL

Hematocrit (HT):

- male, 41% to 53%
- female, 36% to 46%

Mean corpuscular volume (MCV):

- 80 to 100 μm^3

Mean corpuscular hemoglobin (MCH):

- 25.4 to 34.6 pg/cell

Mean corpuscular hemoglobin concentration (MCHC):

- 31% to 36% Hb/cell

Platelets:

- 150,000 to 400,000/mm^3

Endoscopy

Risks to be discussed with a patient prior to endoscopy

A patient consenting to endoscopy needs to be aware of the risks of an adverse reaction to the sedation used, arrhythmia, infection, pain, bleeding, or perforation. Upper endoscopy [esophagogastroduodenoscopy (EGD)] can also lead to aspiration or respiratory depression. Lower endoscopy (colonoscopy, sigmoidoscopy, and enteroscopy) can cause dehydration and an uncomfortable blotting from the gases used during exploration and polyp removal. These risks are greater in those with preexisting conditions such as lung, liver, or cardiac disease. A thorough history and screening for potential problems should be completed and prophylactic intravenous fluids and antibiotics considered.

Urine specimens

Instructions to gather a clean-catch urine specimen

Begin with clean hands.

For females, instruct them to sit on the toilet and spread apart the labia with two fingers. They should then gently cleanse the inner labia, from front to back, twice. Continue to hold open the labia, then begin urinating. Stop the urine flow, and hold the collection container a few inches away from the urethra before beginning the stream of urine again. Only a few inches of urine need to be collected in the specimen cup. Cover and label the specimen clearly.

For males, clean the head of the penis. Retract the foreskin as needed and begin cleaning at the urethral opening and continue down and away from the head of the penis. Begin urinating. Stop the urine flow, and hold the collection container a few inches away from the penis before beginning the stream of urine again. Only a few inches of urine need to be collected in the specimen cup. Cover and label the specimen clearly.

Pathophysiological mechanisms of dyspnea

The vascular bed begins to decrease from thromboemboli, tumor emboli, vascular obstruction, radiation, chemotherapy toxicity, or concomitant emphysema. As the vascular bed decreases, the physiological dead space causes increased ventilation demands. This results in hypoxemia and severe deconditioning with metabolic acidosis, alterations in carbon dioxide output (VCO_2), and arterial partial pressure of carbon dioxide (PCO_2). This also increases neural reflex activity, anxiety, and depression. Inspiratory muscle weakness from cachexia, electrolyte imbalances, neuromuscular abnormalities and steroid use, pleural or parenchymal disease, reduced chest wall compliance, and airway obstruction (such as asthma, tumor growth, and COPD) can produce impaired mechanical responses and ventilatory pump impairment.

Pattern of creatine kinase (CK) following a myocardial infarction (MI)

CK and CK-MB levels are evaluated every 6 to 8 hours in a suspected myocardial injury. Total CK and CK-MB (specific to cardiac cells) initially rise within the first 4 to 6 hours of an MI. A normal range would be 30 IU/L to 180 IU/L for CK and CK-MB totaling 0% to 5% of the CK level.

Assuming no further damage is sustained, peak levels (in excess of six times the normal range) are reached between 12 to 24 hours after the injury.

CK levels will return to normal within 3 to 4 days of the event.
Small spikes in CK level might also occur following invasive cardiac procedures.

Hyperkalemia

A normal potassium level is between 3.5 to 5mEq/L. Elevated potassium, or hyperkalemia, is normally classified as a level greater than 6mEq/L. It is possible to see a false-high potassium level if the blood cells rupture during or after the lab draw. True hyperkalemia is most often caused by impaired kidney function or heavy alcohol or recreational drug use, Addison's disease, type 1 diabetes, severe injury, use of ACE inhibitors, or overuse of potassium supplements. Along with elevated blood potassium levels, the electrocardiogram will show peaked T waves, flattened P waves, prolonged PR interval, and wide QRS complexes. The patient may also complain of muscle fatigue, weakness, partial paralysis, or nausea.

Sleep studies

Sleep study options include the polysomnogram (PSG), multiple sleep latency test (MSLT), maintenance of wakefulness test (MWT), actigraphy, and home-based portable monitoring devices. The PSG test requires an overnight sleep center visit. It monitors bodily functions (electroencephalogram, heart rate, respirations, oxygen level) during sleep in order to identify and properly diagnose sleep-related disorders such as sleep apnea, restless leg syndrome (RLS), and related conditions such as sleep-triggered seizures. Home-based monitoring may be an abbreviated option for extensive PSG studies. The MSLT and MWT are daytime measurements of wakefulness. Actigraphy is a portable, continuous monitoring system of activity levels and sleep patterns. Sleep studies may be considered if a patient mentions having trouble falling asleep or staying asleep, snores, or complains of extreme tiredness and fatigue during most waking hours.

Shock patients

Initial testing for all apparent shock patients

Shock can be classified into several causative categories: hypovolemic, hemorrhagic, cardiogenic, neurogenic, glycemic (hypo- or hyper-), and anaphylactic. Shock is treated as an emergency situation, with the highest priority going toward assessing and maintaining the ABCs (airway, breathing, circulation). While some needed additional information may vary depending on whether or not the type of shock is known, other information is universally gathered. This testing includes vital signs, electrolytes, glucose, urinalysis, serum creatinine, CBC, blood type and match, coagulation studies, pulse oximetry, and blood gases.

Formulating Most Likely Diagnosis

Hyphema

Hyphema refers to the presence of blood in the front area of the eye. This blood is normally the result of mild trauma to the eye. Other causes might include blood vessel abnormalities, infection or inflammation, or ocular cancer. Patients may complain of eye pain, vision changes, and sensitivity to light. In most cases, the blood will be reabsorbed within a few days without treatment of any kind. If natural healing does not occur, the patient may need to undergo intraocular pressure measurement, ultrasound, vision, and glaucoma screenings. Also note a history of sickle cell disease.

Cystocele versus rectocele

When the vaginal wall becomes weakened, a cystocele and/or rectocele results.

When the weakness occurs on the side against the bladder, it is called a cystocele or prolapsed bladder. Muscle weakness can result from straining during childbirth, chronic constipation, coughing, or heavy lifting. Patients might present with complaints of pressure within the vagina; a feeling of discomfort when sitting; pain when bearing down, having intercourse, coughing, or lifting; multiple urinary tract infections; or urine leakage.

A rectocele is a weakness on the posterior wall against the rectum that occurs from the same types of injury. There is a complaint of vaginal fullness, discomfort when sitting, and difficulty passing stool.

Depression

The depressed patient may present with any number of the following: depressed mood; insomnia or hypersomnia; an absence of pleasure in previously enjoyed activities; psychomotor retardation; fatigue; feelings of worthlessness and guilt; and an inability to concentrate, make decisions, or remember important information. The patient may experience significant and unexplained weight loss or weight gain. In severe cases, he or she may also disclose recurrent thoughts of death or suicide. Severity is assigned by the presence of an expressed intent with a plan and means to carry out a suicide attempt, as well as previous attempts. The hallmark symptoms of depression are appetite and sleep changes and decreased energy and concentration. However, in the presence of physical illness, these symptoms can be masked or created by the disease process or corresponding treatments. With preexisting illness, symptoms such as fearfulness, depressed or changed appearance, social withdrawal, brooding, self-pity and pessimism, and a depressed mood or affect that cannot be changed or lifted may be more reliable indicators of depression.

Depression versus seasonal affective disorder

Seasonal affective disorder (SAD) complaints include lethargy, depression, and loss of interest in normal activities that normally manifests in the fall and increase into the winter months then lessen in the spring and summer. Symptoms may be lessened during daylight hours and worsen on dark days and at night. Patients with SAD complain of hopelessness, irritability, increased appetite, and weight gain.

Depression can manifest from substance abuse, medical conditions, medications, prolonged sleep deprivation, and recent stressful life events. It creates a distortion of thought, hopelessness, agitation, irritability, change in thought processes, lethargy, and an extreme change in appetite and sleep patterns.

Both depression and SAD are more common in women than men.

Common medical conditions associated with depression

Patients experiencing depression have a greater tendency toward medical illnesses and vise versa. Underlying causes and links may be found in multiple areas of the assessment. Patients with cardiovascular disease, congestive heart failure, arrhythmias, and heart attacks are prone to a higher incidence of depression. Within the central nervous system cerebrovascular anoxia or accident, Huntington's disease, subdural hematoma, Alzheimer's disease and dementia, human immunodeficiency virus (HIV) infection, carotid stenosis, temporal lobe epilepsy, multiple sclerosis, postconcussion syndrome, myasthenia gravis, narcolepsy, and subarachnoid hemorrhage patients are at increased risk.

Other causes can include rheumatoid arthritis, thyroid disease, diabetes, Cushing's disease, Addison's disease, anemia, lupus, liver disease, syphilis, encephalitis, alcoholism, and general malnutrition.

Tourette syndrome

Tourette syndrome (TS) is a neurological disorder that manifests repetitive, involuntary movements, and vocalizations. These are referred to as tics. Simple tics might include eye movements, grimacing, shrugging, jerking, grunting, throat-clearing, or sniffling. Complex tics are created with combined, coordinated activities, full words, or phrases. These symptoms first appear in the preschool or early elementary school child and are more common in males than females. There is often a worsening of the condition during puberty with a gradual resolution into adulthood. Treatment is not required unless the tics interfere with normal daily functioning. Medication with neuroleptics may then be considered as a means of providing some control.

Galactorrhea

Galactorrhea refers to an abnormal milky discharge from the nipple of one or both breasts that is not related to lactation. It can occur spontaneously or be produced by manual manipulation. Discharge can be continuous or intermittent. This condition is more common in women, but it may occur in men or infants. This condition can be brought on by excessive breast stimulation, side effects of certain medications (hormone supplements, tranquilizers, antidepressants, blood pressure medications, and some herbal supplements), or pituitary gland disorders. Patients presenting with this complaint may also be experiencing dysmenorrhea, headache, or vision changes. If the discharge is other than a milky substance, it may indicate a more significant underlying disease state such as cancer.

Right- and left-sided heart failure

Right-sided heart failure (cor pulmonale) generally results from long-term high blood pressure or chronic lung disease, such as chronic obstructive pulmonary disease (COPD). It is a failure of the right side of the heart to efficiently retrieve blood from the body, and it causes fluid retention. Symptoms can include an activity-dependent altered level of consciousness, complaints of chest pain or discomfort, dependent edema, and altered breathing state (wheezing or cough). Patients may also present with ascites, gastrointestinal complaints, cyanosis, swollen liver, abnormal heart sounds, and neck vein distension. Right-sided heart failure can also result from preexisting left-sided heart failure.

Left-sided heart failure is a result of a dysfunction in the heart's ability to pump blood to the rest of the body correctly (the responsibility of the left ventricle). This causes fluid retention in the lungs (pulmonary edema). The patient may present with cardiomegaly and marked dyspnea.

Paronychia with herpetic whitlow

Herpetic whitlow can form tiny pustules resembling blisters (clear fluid), and their location is further away from the nail bed than paronychia lesions (deeper yellow-green abscess). Herpetic whitlow often affects more than one finger at a time, paronychia is generally focused on one nail bed.

Paronychia is caused by fungus or bacteria with complete resolution with treatment. Herpetic whitlow is a herpes simplex viral infection, which will remain dormant in the body. Herpetic whitlow is not treated by draining the infected area as paronychia often is; herpetic whitlow will often resolve itself.

Aphthous ulcers versus oral herpes

Aphthous ulcers (also known as canker sores) are small, shallow, round or oval lesions occurring inside the mouth. Canker sores are not contagious and are more likely to be the result of injury to the area, malnutrition, or stress. Cold sores (oral herpes) most often occur on the lips, have a more blisterlike appearance, and are highly contagious. Only oral herpes is caused by the herpes virus, which lies dormant within the body and manifests during times of illness or high stress levels. Both conditions can be painful and create difficulties eating, drinking, and talking. Both types of lesions will heal on their own within two weeks.

Diabetes mellitus (DM)

Diabetes mellitus (DM) indicates a patient's difficulties for metabolizing carbohydrates, fat, and proteins with these metabolic changes; the most notable clinical symptom is chronic hyperglycemia. Diabetes mellitus is associated with complications including peripheral vascular disease, coronary artery disease, and diabetic neuropathy. The diabetic patient is also at greater risk for infection and delayed wound healing. Diabetes is also the number one cause for kidney failure. Without conscious and consistent treatment interventions, death can occur at any time.

Diabetes mellitus type 1

Type 1 diabetics have an almost complete loss of insulin production by a functional restriction within the B-cells of the islet of Langerhans located in the pancreas. Restricted insulin production is generally identified in the pediatric patient. Initial symptoms can include weight loss as well as increased thirst, hunger, and urination. Treatment is provided through diet, glucose monitoring, and insulin injections.

Diabetes mellitus type 2

In type 2 diabetes, insulin is available, but the cells have become resistant to it. This condition results in high insulin and glucose levels within the blood as the insulin is unable to transport the glucose effectively. Patient symptoms can be vague or go unnoticed at first. Common complaints can include increased weight, lipid imbalances, and hypertension. Treatment will focus on dietary interventions for weight control, monitoring the blood glucose level, and providing antidiabetic medications. These medications act to inhibit glucose production and increase insulin secretion as well as cell recognition and acceptance of the available insulin.

Esophageal achalasia

Achalasia is a disorder of the esophagus that affects motility. Patients present with dysphagia with both solids and liquids. Other symptoms might include pain, heartburn, cough, or a slight regurgitation of food. Achalasia is most common in middle-aged and older adults. It can also be a genetic trait. Achalasia can be present in esophageal tumors, Zenker diverticulum, Chagas disease, nutcracker esophagus, and diffuse esophageal spasms. Testing includes manometry studies and barium swallow to rule out a mass or tumor. Laboratory results may also show anemia or malnutrition. Treatments can include Botox injections, medications aimed at esophageal sphincter relaxation, esophagogastroduodenoscopy dilatation, or surgery.

Transplant rejection

Hyperacute rejection occurs within minutes to hours of the transplant. This type of reaction occurs when the donated tissue (or blood cells) has not been properly matched to the new host.

Acute rejection happens within days and up to three months after transplant. Acute rejection is the most common form. Most patients will experience at least some degree of acute rejection, and the primary focus of immunosuppressive medication regimes.

Chronic rejection occurs after four months and up to years after the transplant after a slow and constant fight by the body against the tissue that is foreign to the system.

Duodenal and gastric ulcers

Duodenal ulcers are more common than gastric ulcers. The patient often complains of pain relieved by eating. The duodenum secretes bicarbonate to neutralize the hydrochloric acid produced when the patient eats and thus improves the pain. Other symptoms might include increased hunger or feeling of fullness, anemia, blood in the stool, fatigue, and weight loss.

Patients with gastric ulcers present with a history of pain with food. The pain is worse after ingesting food or milk because it stimulates the production of hydrochloric acid, which irritates the stomach ulcer.

Both types are most often caused by *Helicobacter pylori* (*H. pylori*). Definitive diagnosis requires endoscopy.

Viral meningitis

There are approximately 10,000 cases of viral meningitis in the United States each year. Viral meningitis is most common in those younger than five years old or those with compromised immune systems. The most common forms result from infection with enteroviruses, arboviruses, and type 2 herpes simplex virus. Viral meningitis is transmitted through contact with the mentioned viruses, or through contamination with saliva, sputum, mucus, or fecal matter of an already-infected person. The patient presents with fever, nausea, vomiting, light sensitivity, head and neck pain, and a change in mental status. Viral meningitis will often run its course without medical intervention other than monitoring fluids and using universal precautions.

Psoriasis

Psoriasis is a very common, chronic disease affecting 1% to 2% of the United States population. The cause is unknown, but current theories support an autoimmune origin and/or genetics. Psoriasis results from an accelerated skin reproduction cycle. It occurs most frequently on elbows, knees, scalp, intergluteal cleft, penis, and lumbosacral areas. Advanced lesions show abscesses, parakeratotic scales with thinned or absent stratum granulosum. Bacterial and fungal diseases may aggravate psoriasis but are not the primary cause. Other triggers can include stress, skin irritation, sunlight, alcohol consumption, AIDS, chemotherapy, or other autoimmune conditions. Treatment options include creams and ointments, phototherapy, or use of medications such as adalimumab, alefacept, etanercept, infliximab, and stelara.

Bacterial meningitis

Approximately 4,000 cases of bacterial meningitis occur yearly within the United States, resulting in 500 deaths each year. Even in the presence of recovery, there are often lasting consequences of the disease, including brain damage, hearing damage, and learning disabilities. Leading causes include *Haemophilus influenza*, *Streptococcus* strains, *Listeria monocytogenes*, and *Neisseria meningitides.* Contamination results from contact with bacterial-infected saliva, sputum, and mucus. The patient presents with fever, nausea, vomiting, light sensitivity, head and neck pain, and a change in mental status. Immediate treatment with antibiotics is needed. Prevention can also be initiated with vaccination.

Hodgkin disease

Hodgkin disease (Hodgkin lymphoma) is a painless lymphoma in the cervical or supraclavicular region. Palpable nodules in the lymphatic system may be found in the neck, armpits, and groin. The patient may also present with fever, night sweats, weight loss, dry cough, and pruritus. Diagnosis is made by biopsy and identifying the presence of the Reed–Sternberg cell. If caught in the early stages, most cases of Hodgkin disease are curable. It spreads first to other nearby lymph nodes and eventually spreads to the lungs, liver, or bone marrow. Treatment options can include chemotherapy and/or radiation.

Angina pectoris versus myocardial infarction

Angina pectoris often serves as a warning sign for myocardial infarction. Angina is chest pain occurring from reduced blood flow to the myocardium. This pain is described as squeezing, pressure, or burning and is focused on the chest cavity. It is intermittent, often correlating with increased activity and dissipating with rest and/or the use of nitroglycerin. Myocardial infarction occurs when the lack of oxygen perfusion to the heart causes myocardial tissue death. This pain is more extreme, often referred to as crushing, and it extends beyond the chest to radiate out toward the back, shoulder, neck, and jaw. Rest and nitroglycerin will have no effect on this type of pain. Initial treatments will include oxygen and Demerol for pain control. Angina may be diagnosed with an exercise stress test. In the face of a myocardial infarction, an electrocardiogram will show ST changes and laboratory results will show elevated troponin and creatinine levels.

Irritable bowel syndrome versus inflammatory bowel disease

Irritable bowel syndrome (IBS) is the most common intestinal disorder in America. It does not actually affect the actual tissue of the bowel, although there may occasionally be an infection present. The actual cause is unknown, and it occurs in women more than men. The patient may present with complaints of abdominal pain, cramping, bloating, and changes in bowel habits.

Inflammatory bowel disease (IBD) is an actual inflammation or abnormality of the bowel caused by an immune response, such as Crohn's disease or ulcerative colitis. The initial cause is also unknown. Symptoms may include fever, stomach cramps, and bloody diarrhea. Joints, eyes, skin, and liver may also show signs of the disease, and it increases the patient's risk for colon cancer.

Myasthenia gravis

Myasthenia gravis is an autoimmune disorder affecting the neuromuscular system. There is no known cause. Myasthenia gravis causes skeletal muscle weakness by blocking neurotransmitters and interrupting messages from nerve cells to the muscle. Symptoms may worsen with activity and recover with rest. These can include difficulty breathing, chewing, swallowing, talking, performing exertive motions, or controlling eye movements. Other complaints might include fatigue and a change in voice and vision. Testing may show muscle weakness, but no change in reflexes or sensation. Treatment focuses on reducing stress, scheduling activities to allow for rest, and using medications such as neostigmine or pyridostigmine to improve neural communication and prednisone, azathioprine, cyclosporine, or mycophenolate to suppress extreme immune responses.

Cholecystitis

Most cases of acute cholecystitis are caused by gallstones. Cholecystitis pain is most often found in the right upper quadrant. The pain can be described as sharp, cramping, dull, or constant and may radiate to the back or just below the right shoulder blade. The patient may have complaints of pain after eating, but often the pain is delayed by two to four hours. Other symptoms include pale, gray, or clay-colored stools; jaundice; fever; nausea; and vomiting. Further complications might include pus or gangrene in the gallbladder, pancreatitis, or peritonitis. Testing should include complete blood count (CBC), liver function tests, ultrasound, x-ray, and/or computed tomography (CT) scan. Treatments to consider prior to surgery can include antibiotic, a low-fat diet, and pain control.

Graves' disease

Graves' disease is an autoimmune disorder resulting in hyperthyroidism. The hormones secreted by the thyroid are responsible for controlling metabolism. The form of hyperthyroidism caused by Graves' disease is the most common form, often found in women older than age 20. Symptoms and patient complaints can occur in body systems, including: anxiety, nervousness, fatigue, insomnia, changes in mental status, changes in vision, temperature intolerance, amenorrhea, changes in breathing and cardiac patterns, changes in bowel habits, and increased appetite combined with weight loss rather than gain. An enlarged thyroid, or goiter, can often be felt. Laboratory testing should measure TSH, T3, and T4 levels. Ultrasound or CT scan should be used to visualize the thyroid tissue. Treatment options might include antithyroid medications such as methimazole (Tapazole), radiation or surgery.

Gonorrhea and chlamydia

Gonorrhea is a bacterial infection caused by *Neisseria gonorrhoeae* and can be spread through oral, vaginal, penile, or anal contact. Symptoms may appear within two days of infection, but they may be delayed up to a month in men. Female symptoms include vaginal discharge and pain in the lower abdomen/pelvis, with urination and during intercourse. Male symptoms can also include discharge and pain during urination and swollen and tender testicles. Sore throat and fever may also be present.

Chlamydia is a bacterial infection caused by *Chlamydia trachomatis*. Though chlamydia is more common than gonorrhea, it often goes undetected because of minimal symptoms. If symptoms are present, they often mimic those of gonorrhea. Left untreated, infertility can result in women.

Gonorrhea and chlamydia coexist in 50% of cases. Where both conditions exist, the recommended treatment is with doxycycline or azithromycin.

Migraine versus cluster headaches

A migraine is classified as a throbbing headache accompanied by nausea, vomiting, photophobia, and sensitivity to sound that can last for hours or days. The headache may be preceded by a sensory warning, an aura, a smell, a change in vision, or a sensation on the skin. Each patient's sensory warning is unique. There may also be other subtle changes in bowel habits, mental outlook, appetite, and mood in the day or two prior to each episode. Migraines are more common in women.

Cluster headaches are so named because of their tendency to occur in "clusters." Attacks will happen frequently over a few weeks or months and then go into a remission period. There is no defining aura or warning sign of pending attacks. The patient is often awakened in the night to the pain on one side of their head. Cluster headaches are more common in men.

Syphilis

Direct visualization of *Treponema pallidum* is possible by preparing a slide from a specimen taken from the suspect lesion. It is then viewed with direct darkfield microscopy, immunofluorescence, immunoperoxidase, or silver staining. Serologic tests include nontreponemal and treponemal tests. The nontreponemal [Venereal Disease Research Laboratory, (VDRL)] test is best for testing for secondary syphilis. Specific treponemal testing [fluorescent treponemal antibody absorption (FTA-ABS)] can be used for diagnosing secondary and tertiary syphilis.

Pregnant women, men in same-sex relationships, those infected with HIV, or those with partners testing positive for the disease should be screened for syphilis.

Cases of syphilis are reported in every state and tracked by the Centers for Disease Control (CDC).

AIDS infections and malignancies

The AIDS patient is highly susceptible to many bacterial, viral, fungal, and parasitic infections as well as certain types of cancers, such as Kaposi's sarcoma, central nervous system lymphoma, and non-Hodgkin's lymphoma.

Bacterial infections include streptococcus pneumonia, *Mycobacterium avium* intracellulare (MAI) and *Mycobacterium avium* complex (MAC), tuberculosis (TB), salmonellosis, syphilis, and bacillary angiomatosis.

Viral infections include cytomegalovirus (CMV), viral hepatitis, herpes simplex virus (HSV), human papillomavirus (HPV), and progressive multifocal leukoencephalopathy (PML).

Fungal infections include *Candida albicans, Histoplasma capsulatum,* and cryptococcal meningitis.

Parasitic infections include *Pneumocystis carinii* pneumonia (PCP), toxoplasmosis, and cryptosporidium. The rates of contamination with these types of infections in AIDS patients far exceed the rates found within the general population.

Signs and symptoms of leukemia

Leukemia is classified as acute or chronic depending on the type of cell that it originates from and the genetic chromosomal or growth factor deviation present in the malignant cells. Hematological malignancies evolve from immature blood cells multiplying profusely and compromising the integrity of the normal blood cells. Clinical findings can include infection; anemia; fever; and an enlarged liver, spleen, and kidneys accompanied by pain or tenderness over the sternum or other bones and joints. The patient may complain of fatigue, lethargy, and unexplained bleeding and bruising. Further examination may reveal pallor, petechiae, purpura, and bleeding mucous membranes. As normal blood cells become depleted, anemia, infection, and hemorrhage become more common occurrences and can result in death.

Sickle cell disease

Sickle cell disease is one of the most common genetic diseases in the United States, generally affecting those of African, Middle Eastern, Mediterranean, and Indian decent. Sickle cell disease is identified by the signature presence of an abnormal globulin gene, which allows hemoglobin S to form: a "sickle" shape rather than rounded hemoglobin. This sickle shape shortens the lifespan of the hemoglobin causing a chronic anemic state. Pallor, jaundice, weakness, and fatigue are common symptoms. A crisis occurs when the cells clump together causing thrombi and vascular occlusions, leading to hypoxia and even myocardial infarction. It is also associated with multiple acute pain events. Pain episodes are individualized and can vary in both frequency and severity. A sickle cell crisis is identified by pale lips, tongue, palms, or nail beds; lethargy and difficulty awakening; listlessness; irritability; severe pain; or high fever for at least two days. The sickle cell patient is also at higher risk for bacterial infections. Children with sickle cell disease are generally hospitalized less than six times a year. In the patient older than 20 years of age, more than three hospitalizations in a year may be an indication of impending death.

Amyotrophic lateral sclerosis (ALS)

Amyotrophic lateral sclerosis (ALS) is a rapidly progressing muscle degenerative disease with an unknown origin. The main area of involvement is the motor neurons of the brain and spinal cord. Approximately half of patients presenting with ALS will have difficulty swallowing as their first symptom. Other patients will experience distal weakness. As the disease progresses, weakness affects both the upper and lower neurons. Swallowing and oral nourishment are of high concern for these patients. Loss of motility in the tongue and hypopharynx result in the loss of ability to manipulate food as well as creating speech and communication barriers. Death generally results from respiratory failure due to weakness in the diaphragm along with decreased laryngeal and lingual functionality.

Parkinson's disease

Parkinson's disease is a fairly common disease of the central nervous system. There is a slow progression of motor skill complications including resting tremors, excessive slowness in activity, and rigidity. Classic signs include pill-rolling movements in the hands, loss of facial expression, difficulty initiating movements, and gait changes. Because of its slow progression, patients may initially present with generalized weakness, aching, fatigue, and malaise. A slight tremor of an extremity may also be noted. Symptoms result from an imbalance between dopamine-activated and acetylcholine-activated neural pathways in the basal ganglia and are generally found in people older than 65. Parkinson-like symptoms can also be caused by medication toxicity, head trauma, or other degenerative conditions.

Stroke or cerebrovascular accident (CVA)

Within the United States, stroke is the third leading cause of death. A stroke or cerebrovascular accident (CVA) occurs from damage and death of brain cells from clots or plaque within a blood vessel, or the rupture of a vessel. The extent of the damage, including patient death, and the symptoms presented are dependent upon the location and size of the vascular compromise. Common symptoms can include weakness, loss of voluntary movement, paralysis, or a loss of sensation on one side of the body. These conditions can result in other problems such as speech and swallowing problems with increased drooling, as well as impairing the balance and vision and their breathing. If damage is extensive enough, unconsciousness or death can occur.

Assessment tools

All of these assessment tools are used to help determine a patient's overall ability to function in general activities of daily living (ADLs) and review the patient's ease in meeting his or her own needs.
The Karnofsky Performance Scale (KPS) is based on a 0 to 100 scale rating the patient's success in completing his or her own ADLs. Higher scores indicate higher levels of competence with 100 representing full ability without patient complaint. As the numbers decrease, so does the patient's need for outside help with ADLs.
Eastern Cooperative Oncology Group (ECOG) Performance Status uses a 0 to 5 scale as a correlation between the patient's disease process and its effects on his or her own ADL competencies. Lower numbers indicate a lower level of restriction related to the disease process.

The Palliative Performance Scale (PPSv2) rates the patient's abilities in only the following five areas: ambulation, activity, current disease manifestations, self-care, nutritional intake, and level of consciousness. These are rated as a percentage that correlates to their success in these functions.

Dementia

Dementia is defined as a progressive, irreversible state of decline in mental function. The state of dementia is chronic and irreversible. Its onset is quiet and slow. Symptoms do not change over the course of the day. Mental clarity remains intact until the later stages but may be complicated by delirium. Short-term memory may be affected early on, but attention span generally remains intact until later stages. Orientation to person, place, and time remain unaltered until later stages when the person may have difficulty recognizing familiar and common objects (anomia) or recognizing familiar people (agnosia). The patient experiences aphasia, a difficulty finding appropriate words and expressing thoughts clearly. Delusions and hallucinations are most often absent. Psychomotor activity is generally unaffected, but the patient may exhibit signs of apraxia, a difficulty initiating purposeful movement. Sleep and wake cycles become fragmented.

Cirrhosis of the liver

When toxins, inflammation, or metabolic changes within the liver create nodules and fibrosis, cirrhosis is the resulting condition. Cirrhosis of the liver is incurable, although in some cases a liver transplant might be considered as an option. The nodules and fibroids interfere with blood flow through the liver that can cause blood to back up in the spleen. When blood pools within the spleen, it becomes enlarged and blood platelet counts fall. Cirrhosis can also cause gastric and esophageal varices. If not treated, these varices can rupture and bleed, which can result in death. Abdominal ascites and peripheral edema often result from the blood flow restrictions as well. The patient begins to exhibit jaundice coloring in the eyes and then in the skin. Rectal hemorrhoids are also common. Hormonal, metabolic, and kidney disturbances can also result from cirrhosis. Treatment regimens focus on the underlying cause while attempting to slow or halt disease progression, but damage cannot be repaired. Options include abstaining from alcohol use or hepatotoxic drugs. Medications such as prednisone, ursodiol (Actigall), lactulose, and azathioprine (Imuran) can be administered. Diet alterations include low-sodium and low-protein diets with increased vitamin K intake.

Anxiety

Anxiety is marked by feelings of excessive worry, irritability, restlessness, intense feelings of danger, and agitation. The source of the disquiet is unknown or very vague. The patient may have trouble falling or staying asleep and experience interference with other normal activities in their daily lives. Physically, the patient may be identified as having frequent crying spells, headaches, muscle tension, stomach and intestinal distress, palpitations, shortness of breath, anorexia, or overeating. Psychologically, the patient is vulnerable to unrealistic fears and obsessions with harmful ideas and compulsions. Patients may also try to self-medicate with multiple chemicals or substances in attempts to alleviate any of these symptoms. An anxiety disorder is identified by the persistence of these symptoms over a period of six months or more.

Health Maintenance

Hypertriglyceridemia

Management options for hypertriglyceridemia

The main goal of any dietary changes should focus on weight loss because, in the absence of other causative diseases, it is often directly connected to the triglyceride level. A recommendation to limit total fat intake to 10% of the daily calorie consumption and to introduce exercise can often be made. Careful examination of the total LDL and HDL cholesterol levels will help with fine-tuning dietary and exercise recommendations. Testing should also be done to rule out metabolic syndrome. Medication supplements such as statins, fibrates, niacin, and fish oil can also assist in the preventative and recovery process. A referral to a lipidologist or endocrinologist may be needed.

Phenylketonuria

Diet

Phenylketonuria (PKU) causes a buildup of the amino acid phenylalanine, found in protein-based foods, in the blood. Therefore, the main focus of diet recommendations for PKU is on restricting protein intake. General diet restrictions include avoiding milk, eggs, cheese, nuts, beans, soy, chicken, beef, pork, fish, peas, beer, chocolate, and foods containing aspartame. Limits on fruits, vegetables, and simple carbohydrates are also common. Diet, growth, and blood levels of phenylalanine will need to be frequently monitored in order to make adjustments in the individual patient's dietary needs.

Fecal impaction

Fecal impaction happens when it becomes impossible for a hard, dry portion of stool to pass through the rectum. This most often occurs in a patient experiencing chronic constipation who has been using laxatives for extended periods of time, then stops suddenly. The muscles of the intestines and colon have atrophied and can no longer move stool without assistance. Other risk factors include immobility and side effects from medications such as anticholinergics, antidiarrheal agents, and pain medications with methadone or codeine. Treatment options may include manual extraction, suppositories, or surgery. Preventative maintenance includes diet and activity modifications and setting specific parameters for laxative and stool softeners.

Health screenings

Adult female

Although clinical judgment should be used to decide how many, and which, screenings should be focused on for the individual patient, there are common health screenings that should be almost universally provided. Interview questions should include tobacco, alcohol, and recreational drug use; personal safety and abuse; mental health; and personal health beliefs and practices including any alternative health treatments the patient is pursuing. Physical and laboratory assessments should cover hypertension; vision; skin, colon, rectal, cervical and breast cancer screenings; cholesterol; and chlamydia and other sexually transmitted diseases.

Adult male
Though clinical judgment should be used to decide how much and which screenings should be focused on for the individual patient, there are common health screenings that should be almost universally provided. Interview questions should include tobacco, alcohol and recreational drug use, personal safety, mental health, and personal health beliefs and practices including any alternative health treatments the patient is pursuing. Physical and laboratory assessments should cover hypertension, vision, skin, colon, rectal, prostate and testicular cancer screenings, cholesterol, and chlamydia and other sexually transmitted diseases.

Gout

Management options
Treatment for acute episodes includes monitoring water and food intake and medications (pain reliever and anti-inflammatory agents). Gout can be exacerbated by obesity, high blood pressure, impaired kidney function, alcohol, fructose and corn syrup, dehydration, illness, and fever or injury.

Long-term control depends on adequate hydration, weight loss, dietary restrictions (avoidance of alcohol, shellfish, organ and sweets), aerobic exercise, and medications (probenecid, sulfinpyrazone, allopurinol, and febuxostat) to help lower uric acid levels. When medication is being given to control uric acid, monitoring levels through blood testing is essential to find and maintain optimal treatment levels.

Stages of syphilis

Primary syphilis is the first appearance of symptoms: usually a single sore at the point of infection. The lesion is firm, round, and painless and may go unnoticed by the infected individual. The sore(s) heal within three to six weeks with or without treatment, making it even more easily missed.

Secondary syphilis will progress if treatment has not been received and creates a rash on other parts of the body. This rash does not itch. Other symptoms might include fever, swollen lymph nodes, sore throat, hair loss, headache, weight loss, muscle aches, and fatigue.

Latent (late)-stage syphilis is once again a more hidden disease. If the disease process has gone untreated it may appear to resolve on its own, but in reality the infection is moving inward and will show signs of damage to the internal organs (nervous system, circulatory system, bones, joints, and eyes) anywhere from 10 to 30 years after the initial infection.

Diagnostic studies to determine pulmonary embolism

While the best test may be the pulmonary angiogram, it carries more expense and risk than other options that may be considered first.

X ray cannot diagnose pulmonary embolism, but it can rule out other disorders with similar symptoms.

Lung scan measures blood flow in the lungs in the nonsmoker.

Computerized tomography (CT) scan can provide great accuracy in visualizing the lung field.

Magnetic resonance imaging (MRI) has even greater accuracy with a comparable raise in expense, but without the effects of the contrast dye used in the CT scan.

Ultrasound pulses and echocardiogram may also be helpful, as well as a D-dimer blood test to detect the clot.

Somogyi effect

In the diabetic, the Somogyi effect is the body's tendency to overreact to low blood sugar levels. This overcompensation with glucagon and epinephrine to communicate to the liver to convert glycogen stores into readily available glucose creates a new spike in the blood sugar. This phenomenon most often occurs as a result of nighttime hypoglycemia that goes untreated. If a patient is consistently awakening with elevated blood glucose levels, they may need to wake up in the middle of the night in order to perform another blood sugar reading. Their evening intake and insulin dose can then be adjusted to prevent further episodes.

Risks associated with cardiovascular disease

Risk factors that the patient and his or her healthcare provider can exercise some control over are identified as modifiable. These can include smoking; excess weight; alcohol use; cholesterol levels; blood pressure; and active management of diabetes, stress, and the amount of exercise the patient engages in. Risk factors beyond the patient's control include age, male sex, and genetic tendencies including race (Caucasian, black, or Native American) and family history. The greatest risk is to those who have already experienced a cardiovascular event, or have been previously diagnosed with a cardiac vascular disease such as peripheral vascular disease, aortic aneurysm, or carotid artery disease. Others with high risk include those who have at least two of the modifiable or nonmodifiable risk factors or type 2 diabetes.

Management and maintenance of major depression

Medication and therapy are normally needed in order to begin resolving major depression. It is important to note the differences in the amount of time it may take for these approaches to work, however. The patient, especially, needs to understand that their progress may seem slow. Selective serotonin reuptake inhibitors (SSRIs) take between two and six weeks to reach a therapeutic level and should not be adjusted until after that time. Tricyclic antidepressants (TCAs) can also take several weeks and carry an increased risk of adverse effects. Monoamine oxidase inhibitors (MAOIs) should not be combined with SSRIs. There should be a cleansing period of four to five weeks between administration of SSRI and MAOIs. Other treatments that may be considered include light therapy, transcranial magnetic stimulation (TMS), or electroconvulsive therapy (ECT). The patient should also be advised that alcohol and recreational drug use can feed the problem rather than provide the relief they are seeking.

AIDS dementia complex (ADC)

The exact cause of AIDS dementia complex (ADC) is unknown, but it is a primary result of the disease process itself. Current theories suggest that the HIV infection stimulates an invasion of macrophages in the brain (microglia). These release cytokines that directly damage the nervous tissue by disrupting the neurotransmitter functions and causing encephalopathy. This condition affects as many as 15% of all AIDS patients. Prognosis is poor, and the disease is not reversible. However, retroviral drugs can delay its onset. Central nervous system HIV infections in children tend to have a more dramatic and pronounced effect than those occurring in adults. ADC is characterized by gradual memory loss, decreased concentration and cognition, as well as mood disorders. The patient may also experience physical symptoms of ataxia, incontinence, and seizures.

Osteoporosis

Osteoporosis describes bones that have become weak, brittle, and prone to fractures from even mild stress. Early signs and symptoms may include complaints of back pain, diminished height, hunched or stooped posture, and eventual fracture that occurs from what otherwise would have been considered a minor injury.
Postmenopausal Caucasian and Asian women carry the greatest risk for developing osteoporosis. Diagnosis is made through measuring bone density with dual-energy x-ray absorptiometry (DXA). Therapy often includes the prescription of bisphosphonates (alendronate, risedronate, ibandronate, or zoledronic acid). Hormone replacement therapy (HRT) after menopause can help prevent osteoporosis. Prevention counseling might also include weight-bearing exercise, smoking cessation, minimal alcohol consumption, and guidance in safe environments and practices to avoid falls.

Implications of kidney failure

When the kidneys become unable to function either short- or long-term, it is referred to as kidney failure. Causes for kidney failure may include toxins such as some medications, tumors, infections, diabetes, hypertension, and collagen vascular diseases such as lupus. When there is hope of restoring normal kidney function, peritoneal dialysis or hemodialysis as well as diuretics and the treatment of underlying causes such as hypertension can be used. Dietary treatments focus on managing the patient on a low-sodium, low-protein, and low-potassium diet. Dialysis, and its supplementary treatments, is also the treatment for chronic kidney failure. However, when there is no hope of return to normal kidney function, the patient faces the difficult decisions of whether or not to start, continue, or even stop the dialysis. These decisions will either prolong the patient's life or bring death within just a few days. As the disease progresses, it brings more pronounced complications in fluid and electrolyte balances, anemia, and uremia. At this point, the patient's treatment may turn to focus on comfort and medications rather than prolonged life by use of dialysis.

Education for the patient with acute or chronic illnesses

Diagnosis: Establish a basic understanding of the disease process, including areas of the body affected, causes, prognosis, and whether or not it is contagious.

Complications: Clarify possible signs and symptoms, early warning signs, and signals to disease progression and healing

Management: Define what the patient can expect from his care and recovery, including treatments, diet, activity levels, and medications.
Aggravating factors: Help the patient understand what behaviors or triggers may increase his symptoms and what can be done to avoid or control them.

Prognosis: Patients need both an immediate idea of what to expect as well as a long-term picture of what to expect.

Prevention: Establish self-care habits that can help prevent reoccurrence of the problem.

Resources: Make sure the patient is informed of all available resources to help him on his healthcare journey.

Ages of childhood immunizations

Birth: Hepatitis B (Hep B)

1-2 Months: Hep B; rotavirus vaccine (RV); diphtheria, tetanus, pertussis (DTaP); *Haemophilus Influenzae* type B (Hib); pneumococcal conjugate vaccine (PCV); inactivated polio vaccine (IPV)

4 Months: RV, DTaP, Hib, PCV, IPV

6 Months: Hep B, RV, DTaP, Hib, PCV, IPV

12-18 Months: Hep B; DTaP; Hib; PVC; IPV; measles, mumps, rubella (MMR); varicella; hepatitis A (Hep A)

4-6 Years: DTaP, IPV, MMR, varicella

11-12 Years: DTaP, human papillomavirus (HPV), meningococcal conjugate vaccine (MCV4)

Environmental factors that affect the severity of asthma

Common environmental triggers for asthma exacerbation include seasonal allergies created by pollen, weather patterns, mold spores, animal dander, smoke, smog, other odors such as perfumes, and household and cleaning chemicals. Exposure to things such as dust mites during infancy can even be a key factor in the initial development of asthma. Other factors to consider include hormone fluctuations, exercise, foods, and medications used for other conditions (NSAIDs and beta-blockers). Any effort made to control or remove known triggers creates positive results for overall lung heath as well as the number of acute asthma attacks.

Impacts of stress on health

Excessive stress occurs when the body's natural "fight-or-flight" instinct becomes overstimulated. This creates an overload of adrenaline, cortisol, and glucose in the system and reduces the function of body systems not needed for immediate response to a crisis. Stress alters the immune, cardiac, digestive, and reproductive systems. It increases the patient's risk for heart disease, sleep disorders, skin disorders, digestive problems, altered thought processes including memory and emotion, tobacco, alcohol and drug abuse, obesity, and autoimmune disorders as well as exacerbating these conditions once they exist.

Warning signs and clues indicative of abuse and/or neglect

Regular screening for domestic violence in a healthcare setting is a helpful and inoffensive method of identifying victims. Watch for injuries that do not seem to match the story given. Overbearing or overprotective partners who answer for or dominate your interview with the patient, frequent nonspecific complaints such as headache, stomach, neck and back pain, insecurity, stammering or avoidance in giving responses to simple questions, intestinal complaints, and sexually transmitted disease. In the abused adolescent female tobacco, alcohol and drug use, decreased school attendance, isolation, and bulimia are more common.

National Environmental Public Health Tracking program

The National Environmental Public Health Tracking (EPHT) program was designed by the Centers for Disease Control (CDC) in response to a need for a way to accurately record and analyze the correlations between environmental factors and health trends to help in finding ways to prevent diseases such as poisoning, birth defects, developmental disabilities, cancer, and neurologic and respiratory diseases. Information is gathered through biomonitoring (measurements of how much of various chemicals are actually absorbed into the body) from local, state, and federal agencies as well as academic institutions and other nongovernment organizations. The collected data can be accessed through the CDC.

Clinical Intervention

Sick sinus syndrome

Sick sinus syndrome is most common in the patient older than age 50. It is represented by a pattern of irregular sinus bradycardia with long pauses in conduction. There may also be an accelerated atrial rate or a pattern of bradycardia–tachycardia as the heart tries to correct its rhythm. There are often no clear symptoms, but vague complaints that could mimic other disorders may be seen. These might include angina or a feeling of fluttering or "wrongness" in the chest, a change in mental status, altered consciousness, dizziness, fatigue, and shortness of breath with exertion. Treatment may not be needed if the patient is nonsymptomatic. Permanent treatment is provided by an internal pacemaker, and the associated surgical risks should be discussed with the patient.

Thrombotic thrombocytopenic purpura

Thrombotic thrombocytopenic purpura is classified as a blood disorder with the formation of multiple blood clots and a low platelet count. The first line of treatment is plasma exchange, in which the patient's own plasma is removed and replaced with healthy plasma from a matching donor through transfusion. More than one plasma exchange may be needed to see improvement. If the disease remains unresponsive to this treatment, immunosuppressive medications may be prescribed and a splenectomy can be anticipated.

Seizures

Treatment options

Medication: In many cases, seizures can be effectively controlled with medications such as carbamazepine, ethosuximide, felbamate, tiagabine, levetiracetam, lamotrigine, pregabalin, gabapentin, phenytoin, topiramate, and oxcarbazepine.

Ketogenic diet: A strict diet intended to induce a long-term starvation effect in order to burn ketones may be tried in the child whose seizures aren't easily controlled by medication. This diet is high in fat and low in carbohydrates and requires careful monitoring.
Alternative medicine: Biofeedback, melatonin, and folic acid supplements may also be helpful.

Surgery: Depending on the type and severity, surgery may sometimes be considered.

Cryptococcosis

Treatment options

Cryptococcosis is a result of a respiratory fungal infection by *Cryptococcus neoformans*. This condition is most often found among those with compromised immune systems. Mild cases may only require monitoring to ensure that the infection does not spread. In more advanced cases, the infection is treated with antifungal medications such as amphotericin B, flucytosine, and fluconazole. The patient should also be monitored for central nervous system infection and significant side effects caused by the medications.

Cryptorchidism

An undescended testicle (cryptorchidism) is a common occurrence in preterm infants. If the testicle hasn't descended by the time the child is one year old, it should be evaluated and watched. Some testicles will descend and then temporarily retract again. This condition is not true cryptorchidism. Cryptorchidism is linked with decreased fertility and cancer (of both testicles). Injections with the hormone beta human chorionic gonadotropin (B-hCG) or testosterone may help the testicle descend. If this does not work, surgery is the next option.

Pancreatic cancer

Tumor growth may begin without any symptoms and therefore go undetected for an extended period of time. The earliest symptoms include dark urine, clay-colored stools, fatigue, jaundice, changes in appetite, weight loss, and pain in the stomach.

Physical exam may show a positive Courvoisier sign: the presence of a palpable head tumor that can feel like an enlarged gallbladder. Diagnostic testing includes a computed tomography (CT) scan of the abdomen. The Whipple procedure (pancreaticoduodenectomy) and chemoradiation are used for treatment. However, the median survival rate is only 9 to 12 months.

Trichomoniasis and its treatment

Trichomoniasis is a sexually transmitted disease that presents with large amounts of foul-smelling, yellow-green vaginal discharge. This discharge is often described as foamy or frothy. The patient may complain of mild itching or irritation. A wet-mount microscopic specimen will show protozoan flagellate motile organisms. The treatment of choice for the patient with trichomoniasis, and all sexual partners, is with metronidazole. Clotrimazole may be substituted when the disease presents in the first trimester of pregnancy.

Health belief model

The health belief model is a theory framework that helps define how likely an individual is to make or maintain positive health choices. Adherence to any treatment regime is based on the patient's belief that their disease is serious and threatening to their well-being. Action is determined by cues to action, perceived benefits of action, and reduced barriers to action. In order to promote change, the individual, or group's, core motivations and beliefs must be identified and promoted. It is not a system of negative reinforcement or scare tactics but a way to promote positive internal attitude changes toward positive health outcomes.

Initial prenatal consultation

Routine information to gather during a prenatal visit includes weight and blood pressure, urinalysis for occult blood, glucose and bacteria, fundal height, and fetal heart tones after 10 weeks' gestation. Blood work should include type and antibody screening, complete blood count (CBC), rapid plasma reagin, hepatitis B antigen, HIV, and rubella. After 14 weeks, a maternal serum alpha-fetoprotein level can also be obtained. Pap smear and screening for sexually transmitted diseases are also performed. Feelings and expectations regarding pregnancy are explored, and careful questions regarding personal safety and abuse may be proposed. Smoking, alcohol, and recreational drug use should also be addressed.

Hypertension in the diabetic patient

Because of the higher risk for nephropathy, myocardial infarction, and stroke associated with diabetes, it is highly important to adequately treat hypertension. The first line of defense is angiotensin-converting enzyme (ACE) inhibitors; the next choice would be angiotensin II receptor blockers (ARBs), although multiple antihypertensives may be needed. Diuretics are often needed as well.

Outside of medication, the diabetic patient should be encouraged to keep their blood sugar levels under tight control, lose weight as needed, exercise, and quit smoking. All of these will help mitigate the patient's increased risk for atherosclerosis and high blood pressure.

Smoking cessation options

Nicotine dependence is the most common addiction in the United States. The first intervention is simply to begin a conversation with the patient and assess their interest and history of quitting attempts. Counseling, behavioral modification therapy, and one-on-one support can be offered from various sources, but medication may be needed. Nicotine replacement therapy is safe for most patients. Over-the-counter options include nicotine patch, gum, and candy). Prescription options include nicotine inhalers and nasal spray. Non-nicotine medications that may also be helpful include bupropion SR and varenicline. Clonidine and nortriptyline may be considered but are not currently FDA approved and carry many more side effects.

Roles of HDL, LDL, and triglyceride levels in cardiac health

Normal cholesterol and triglyceride results are as follows: total cholesterol—less than 200 mg/dL, HDL—above 60 mg/dL, LDL—below 120 mg/dL, and triglycerides—less than 150 mg/dL.

Low-density lipoprotein (LDL) represents the "bad" cholesterol that is responsible for sticking to the blood vessels to create atherosclerosis. LDL increases heart disease risk.

High-density lipoprotein (HDL) represents "good" cholesterol that helps to remove buildup from the vessel walls. Higher levels of HDL can help reduce the risk of heart disease caused by LDL.

Triglyceride level correlation is still unclear, but elevated levels are linked with an increased risk of heart disease, especially in conjunction with elevated LDL levels.

Skin lesions

Papule—small, solid, raised lesion no larger than 1 cm. Coloring may be brown, purple, red, or pink.

Macule—small (less than 1 cm) discolored spot that is neither raised nor depressed against the surrounding skin. A macule also does not affect the skin texture.

Vesicle—small (5 to 10 mm), elevated, fluid-filled, circular lesion that generally ruptures easily then dries to a yellow crust.

Plaque—wide, large, well-demarcated, plateaulike, elevated lesion that appears red with silvery scaling. Often associated with psoriasis.

Bulla—large (greater than 5 mm), elevated, clear fluid-filled, circular lesion.

Precautions

<u>Purpose and parameters of universal precautions</u>
Universal precautions are designed to promote a reasonable amount of safety for the patient and provider in any caregiving situation. It emphasizes the belief that every patient is a carrier of an infectious agent such as hepatitis B or HIV. Universal precaution requires protective barriers (gloves, gowns, mask, and/or goggles) when there is any chance of coming in contact with blood; semen; and vaginal, synovial, spinal, pleural, peritoneal, amniotic, and pericardial fluids.

<u>Conditions that would require contact precautions</u>
Airborne precautions apply to tuberculosis, chicken pox, shingles, and measles. Doors must remain closed, respirators must be worn at all times within the room, and strict hand-washing procedure is observed.

Contact and enteric precautions apply to cases of antibiotic-resistant infections [methicillin-resistant *Staphylococcus aureus* (MRSA) and vancomycin-resistant enterococci (VRE)], respiratory syncytial virus (RSV), diphtheria, herpes, impetigo, abscesses and skin ulcerations, pediculosis, scabies, staphylococcal furunculosis, zoster, *Clostridium difficile,* and *Escherichia coli.* Gown and gloves are required within the room as well as strict hand-washing procedure.

Droplet precautions apply to meningitis, pneumonia, epiglottitis, pneumonia, bacteremia, group A streptococcal pharyngitis, influenza, scarlet fever, adenovirus, mumps, rubella, and parvovirus B19. This requires a simple mask and strict hand-washing procedure.

Ways a sterile field may be compromised

A sterile field does not extend below the table or platform it is set up on. Contamination can occur if anything below this level comes in contact with the field (such as the sterile gown below the waist level or a portion of the sterile drape folding over the edge of the table touches the field), hands dropped below the level of the table, arms three inches above the wrist, and the back of the sterile gown are also considered contaminated. Sneezing or coughing over the field is contaminating as is replacing an implement in the field that has been transported out of the field or dropped. Fields that are established on a moist surface are considered contaminated. So is a field that is left unattended, uncovered, or has been completely turned away from during a procedure.

Discharge planning

Discharge planning is a formal process that allows care providers to coordinate the individual needs of the patient extending beyond their time in a hospital or long-term-care setting. This assessment process examines how to provide the appropriate provider care once they no longer meet criteria for hospitalization. Also considered is an understanding of the patient's insurance and benefit coverage to ensure that needed services will be available without unreasonable financial burden. The patient must receive clear and accurate teaching about their condition and self-care as well as community resources that will be available to them.

Heartburn

Treatment options

Medication options include antacids (Maalox, Mylanta, Rolaids, and Tums) to neutralize stomach acid; however, long-term use can result in changes in bowel habits. H_2-receptor blockers (Tagamet HB, Pepcid AC, Zantac, and Axid AR) are meant to reduce the stomach's production of acid. Relief isn't as instant as with antacids, but it will last longer. Proton pump inhibitors (Prevacid 24HR and Prilosec) can both reduce acid production and heal the trauma caused to the esophagus. Patient counseling should include weight loss, if needed; avoidance of tight clothing; specific trigger foods; eating smaller, more frequent meals; smoking cessation; and remaining upright after eating.

Options available for cancer treatment

There are three main types of cancer treatment available: surgery, radiation, and chemotherapy. These may be used alone or in combination.

Surgery attempts to remove the entire tumor as well as surrounding tissues that may have been affected in order to produce a curative/cancer-free state in the patient. When this is not possible, surgery can be used as a palliative effort to remove as much of the tumor as possible in order to lessen the associated pain and symptoms for the patient.

Radiation therapy provides localized cancer treatment focusing on the removal of cancer cells before they produce clinical symptoms. Radiation can also be palliative, or used in the treatment of medical emergencies such as spinal cord compression or superior vena cava syndrome.

Chemotherapy uses medications to target and help destroy cancer cells. This therapy can be used alone but it is often combined with other treatments for either a curative objective or palliative focus on symptom and pain control.

Complementary and alternative medicine

As defined by the National Center for Complementary and Alternative Medicine (NCCAM)

Biologically based practice: Focuses on the use of naturally occurring substances and diet for health promotion.

Energy medicine: Asian-based energy and magnetic and biofield beliefs such as Reiki and Qi Gong.

Manipulative and body-based practice: The practice of manipulating body parts or systems as a way to improve or manipulate their performance, such as chiropractic, message, and reflexology.

Mind–body medicine: Focuses on the way mental outlook and belief systems affect health, promoting relaxation and meditation techniques.

Whole medical systems: More conventional medicine working in conjunction and harmony with a specific cultural belief system such as traditional Chinese medicine.

Patient care

<u>Interpersonal and communication skills for quality patient care</u>
The ability to establish a therapeutic relationship with appropriate boundaries.

- Effective and tolerant listening skills as well as the ability to correctly interpret nonverbal cues.
- An understanding of open-ended and guided questions and interview skills.
- Clear and concise writing and documentation skills.
- Comfort and confidence in communicating with individuals from all walks of life.
- Appropriately accommodate messages to optimize understanding in the recipient.
- Remain level-headed and emotionally stable, even in disruptive or contentious situations.
- Able to maintain strict patient confidentiality.

Status epilepticus

Status epilepticus is a seizure lasting longer than five minutes, or the state of repeated seizures without a subsequent return to consciousness, or return of normal brain function, between each separate episode. Status epilepticus is considered to be an emergency. Treatment for status epilepticus focuses on maintaining a clear airway, protecting the patient from eminent harm, and administering medication in an attempt to resolve the episodes. Assess for adequate patient perfusion, give a glucose solution, evaluate the electrolytes, and administer IV benzodiazepines followed by IV phenytoin. Lorazepam is generally the first line of defense; however, if the seizure does not respond to treatment within the first five to seven minutes, phenytoin or fosphenytoin should be added. In extreme cases, barbiturates, anesthesia, neuromuscular blocks, and propofol may be needed to control seizure activity.

Making successful lifestyle and health changes

Change begins with the patient making a firm, concrete commitment to a goal or positive outcome. No change can be achieved without a decision to pursue that change.

Goals that are measurable, gradual, and within the realistic reach for the patient must be established. A clear path needs to be visualized.

A realistic view of negative life events and relapses must be established that allows the patient to be forgiving of their perceived failures and maintain long-term resolve toward the change.

The patient must receive support and encouragement from outside sources that they trust and value.

Collaboration and coordination among healthcare team members

Tools developed for this specific purpose in a healthcare setting include practice guidelines to help define each participant's role in care and clinical protocol or pathway to focus care and clarify procedure and strategies to be followed. The goal is to create a team in which the members understand their own, and each other's, role within the group; understand the goals of the team; share responsibility; reach collective decisions; and actively include the patient and his family in the care process. An effective collaboration effort includes all stages of care, from assessment of needs, action, communication, and evaluation of goals upon completion. A primary key is streamlined communication and respect for each individual's unique contribution. The nurse often plays a primary role as mediator and advocate for the patient, making sure he or she understands the purposes and joint goal of the group and its members.

Risk factors associated with cardiovascular disease

Risk factors that the patient and his or her healthcare provider can exercise some control over are identified as modifiable. These can include the following: smoking, excess weight, alcohol use, cholesterol levels, blood pressure, active management of diabetes, stress, and the amount of exercise the patient engages in.

Risk factors beyond the patient's control include the following: age, male sex, and genetic tendencies including race (Caucasian, black, or Native American) and family history.

The greatest risk is to those who have already experienced a cardiovascular event or those who have been previously diagnosed with a cardiac vascular disease such as peripheral vascular disease, aortic aneurysm, or carotid artery disease. Others with high risk include those who have at least two of the modifiable or nonmodifiable risk factors or type 2 diabetes.

Four types of subacute care facilities

General—patients discharged to this level of care are stable and healing well but still require skilled care for such things as long-term intravenous treatments.

Chronic—chronic care facilities are for terminal and end-of-life patients that cannot be cared for in an at-home setting because of choice or complexity of care such as ventilator dependency.

Transitional—at this level, the patient still needs complex medical and nursing care, such as deep-wound management.

Long-term transitional—identifies a need for continued complex medical care that is expected to have an extended treatment time.

Pulmonary embolism

<u>Findings and treatment priorities</u>

Pulmonary embolism is the second leading cause of sudden death. Immediate recognition and treatment for pulmonary embolism is crucial to the patient's chances of survival. Symptoms can be vague and nonspecific but might include chest pain, dyspnea, tachypnea, cough, abnormal lung sounds, low blood pressure, or even just a sense of impending doom or nonspecific agitation. Pulmonary angiography or computed tomography (CT) angiography is used to make a positive diagnosis. Priority care is given to basic life functions, including monitoring oxygen saturation levels and administering oxygen as needed. Anticoagulants and thrombolytics may be used to dissolve the clot, or it may need to be surgically removed. Nitroglycerin, angiotensin-converting enzyme (ACE) inhibitors, and loop diuretics may also be administered. A vein filter may also be inserted to prevent further clots from reaching the lungs.

Most common nonpain complaints of patients with terminal illnesses

Patients with cancer often express fatigue and anorexia as the top two reasons for emotional and physical distress. Nausea, constipation, states of delirium or other alterations of mental status, and dyspnea are also frequent. Fatigue encompasses symptoms of tiredness, a lack of energy not related to the amount of rest the patient is getting, diminished mental capacity, and weakness. These symptoms interfere with the ability to perform activities of daily living and are often underdiagnosed or downplayed by the patient as inevitable. Anorexia and cachexia are associated with the general wasting of many terminal illnesses and requires careful nutritional management. Nausea and constipation are often related to medications and other treatments but are easily treated if assessed and planned for. Palliative treatments are helpful for altered mental states and dyspnea as well if they are assessed and planned for.

Pharmaceutical Therapeutics

Nystatin

Nystatin (Mycostatin, Nadostine, Nilstat, Nystex) can be used to treat oral candidiasis (thrush) in children and adults as an oral suspension or lozenges at a dose of 200,000 to 600,000 units four times a day for up to two weeks. For treatment of intestinal candidiasis as oral tablets 400,000 to 600,000 units of nystatin is given, up to three times a day. For treatment of vaginal candidiasis, nystatin in the form of vaginal suppositories or tablets of 100,000 units is given up to twice a day for two weeks. Adverse reactions might include nausea, vomiting, stomach discomfort, diarrhea, rash, or vaginal irritation.

Colchicine

Colchicine (Colcrys) is prescribed for gout. Its function is to counteract the swelling and pain from uric acid build up. The normal dosage level is 0.5 to 0.6 mg daily. For acute attacks, an initial dose of up to 1.2 mg can be given, followed by 0.5 to 1.2 mg up to every hour until relief is reached. The intravenous dosage is 2 mg then 0.5 mg every 6 hours with a maximum 24-hour dose of 4 mg. Nausea, vomiting, stomach discomfort, and diarrhea are common reactions. Vitamin B_{12}, alcohol, and grapefruit can interfere with the action of colchicine.

Combantrin

Combantrin (pyrantel pamoate) is an anthelmintic used for treatment of infections caused by parasitic worms such as roundworm and pinworm. Normal dosage is 11 mg/kg (maximum of 1 g) orally, followed by a second dose after two weeks. It is important to treat all family members and others who have close contact with the infected individual and emphasize fastidious personal hygiene habits. Piperazine salts should not be used during the time of treatment, and caution should be used when treatment in needed in patients will severe malnutrition, anemia, or liver impairment.

Minoxidil

Oral minoxidil (Loniten): Loniten is an antihypertensive used in adult patients with severe high blood pressure. Therapeutic dosages must be built up to and usually range from 10 to 40 mg a day. It may cause edema, tachycardia, or other cardiac side effects. Loniten should not be used with NSAIDs or the herb ma huang because they interfere with its action.

Topical minoxidil (Rogaine): Rogaine is a hair growth stimulant available in 2% and 5% topical solutions. These solutions can be applied to areas of thinning hair up to twice a day. Patients should be educated about the possibility of skin irritation and what to expect for results. About 40% of patients will begin to see moderate hair growth after four months of use.

Opiate abuse and withdrawal symptoms

Opioid analgesic therapy is a widely used method of chronic pain control. The severity of symptoms is dependent on the amount and duration of use. Common side effects of abuse may mimic the flu and include increased respirations, diarrhea, runny nose, sweating, coughing, lacrimation, muscle twitching, and increased temperature and blood pressure. Withdrawal symptoms will overlap with abuse symptoms and become worse. Agitation, anxiety, nausea and vomiting, chronic goose bumps, and dilated pupils are also present.
Overdose is treated with naloxone. Withdrawal symptoms can be eased with methadone.

Acetaminophen

Acetaminophen is a non-narcotic analgesic for mild to moderate pain and fever. This pain relief effect can be enhanced when combined with caffeine. Likewise, when acetaminophen is combined with narcotics, it can enhance the pain relief quality of the narcotic. Acetaminophen has no effect on inflammation. It can be safely used in children. It also does not affect blood clotting time. Those with a history of heavy alcohol use should use it cautiously because the combination of the two has a greater chance of creating damage to the liver.

Aspirin

Aspirin is a salicylate analgesic for mild to moderate pain and fever reduction. Use in children is not recommended because of an increased risk of Reye syndrome. Aspirin is also often used as a prophylactic to reduce the risk of myocardial infarction, stroke, and transient ischemic attacks (TIAs) because of its blood thinning quality. It is beneficial in treating inflammation. However, aspirin can also decrease the reabsorption of uric acid, increase gastric irritation, and increase risk of occult blood loss.

Methyldopa

Methyldopa (Aldomet, Aldopren, Dopamet) is an antihypertensive that can be administered orally or by IV. IV dosing is 250 to 500 mg every 6 hours. Oral maintenance dose is 500 mg to 2 g in two or four equal doses. In long-term use, it is often recommended that this medication be taken at bedtime because of its tendency to cause sedation. Other common side effects are headache, orthostatic hypotension, nasal congestion, and dry mouth. Use cautiously with amphetamines, beta-blockers, norepinephrine, phenothiazines, tricyclic antidepressants, anesthesia, barbiturates, haloperidol, levodopa, lithium, MAO inhibitors, and tolbutamide. Monitor blood pressure and liver function closely.

Potassium-sparing diuretics

Potassium-sparing diuretics include amiloride, triamterene, spironolactone, and eplerenone. They are used to prevent sodium reabsorption and potassium secretion in the collection tubules while still promoting urinary excretion of excess fluid. Potassium-sparing diuretics are often used in conjunction with antihypertensive medications to manage high blood pressure or congestive heart failure. Although this class of medications can help prevent hypokalemia, potassium levels still need to be monitored and they should not be used at the same time as potassium supplements.

Common occupational health hazards

The most common accidents to occur in the workplace involve system and mechanical failures. Musculoskeletal complaints such as back pain accompany heavy lifting and repetitive activities. Injuries can be to large muscles (such as the back) or smaller muscle groups (wrists, neck, ankles).

Hearing loss is common in construction and manufacturing industries.

Chemical and biological agents that can cause liver damage, reproductive disorders, and cancer are most common in professions that have constant exposure to pesticides, heavy metal, and corrosive substances.

Healthcare workers are particularly vulnerable to HIV, tuberculosis, and hepatitis B and C.

Mild to moderate acne

Over-the-counter options include lotions containing benzoyl peroxide, sulfur, resorcinol, or salicylic acid. These products are best for mild cases of acne. For more severe cases, the strength of the lotions can be increased through the prescription of tretinoin, adapalene or tazarotene. Beyond topical agents, antibiotics (tetracycline or clindamycin) can be considered as well as oral contraceptives. Chemical peels, microdermabrasion, and laser and light therapy can also be useful. Isotretinoin (Amnesteem, Claravis, Sotret) is an extremely powerful medication, which, while highly effective for scarring cystic acne, carries many risks and side effects and should be considered as a last resort.

COPD

Chronic obstructive pulmonary disease (COPD) cannot be cured, but it can be controlled with medication. Inhalers can be coupled with anti-inflammatory medications. The first line of defense is usually recommended as ipratropium and albuterol (beta-2-adrenergics and anticholinergics), the second-line option is albuterol, and the third choice would be methylprednisolone sodium succinate, followed by theophylline. Acute flare-ups may also require assistance from steroids, nebulizers with bronchodilators, oxygen therapy, and breathing assistance through aids such as a BiPAP portable ventilator. Other recommendations for the patient might include weight management, pulmonary rehabilitation, and reducing triggers in their environment such as smoke or perfumes. Surgery to remove severely damaged lung tissue may also be considered.

Levothyroxine sodium

Considerations for dosing must include patient age, duration and severity of hypothyroidism, and presence of any preexisting cardiac disease such as angina. There is a high level of sensitivity to thyroid medications, so the initial dose should begin at a very low level, generally 25 mcg a day, increasing as needed every one to two months in order to reach therapeutic levels. Adults older than age 60 will require less medication than a younger adult. Levothyroxine increases cardiac workload and elevates heart rate—the patient should inform you of any chest pain, palpitations, sweating, anxiety, or shortness of breath.

Chronic, stable angina

Initial medication choices include beta-blockers such as metoprolol in order to lower the heart rate, blood pressure, and oxygen requirements of the heart. Long-acting nitrates including isosorbide dinitrate may be considered if beta-blockers prove ineffective, but there is a tendency to develop a tolerance to these medications. Ranolazine is also a good choice. Angiotensin-converting enzyme (ACE) inhibitors lower blood pressure. Calcium-channel blockers help the heart relax to reduce workload and blood pressure. Preventive measures against myocardial infarction may also be considered using aspirin, clopidogrel, or prasugrel.

Cystitis

Cystitis is most often caused by *Escherichia coli* (*E. coli*). The patient presents with urinary frequency, urgency, and pain, and there may also be a pain response to light pressure on the suprapubic area. Urinalysis will show white and red blood cells. Because of the increase in strains of *E. coli* that are resistant to trimethoprim-sulfamethoxazole, a three-day course of fluoroquinolones such as ciprofloxacin has now become the standard treatment of choice. These recommendations change frequently according to the mutations of the bacterial strains and should be frequently revalidated in a dependable resource such as *The Sanford Guide to Antimicrobial Therapy*.

Warfarin versus heparin

Warfarin (Coumadin) is an anticoagulant normally given in oral form (2 to 10 mg a day) as long-term therapy for those patients needing blood thinners. This requires both baseline and frequent prothrombin time (PT) and international normalized ratio (INR) levels to maintain a therapeutic level. The patient should also be monitored for unusual bruising and bleeding as well as cautioned against aspirin use and other over-the-counter supplements that affect bleeding times.

Heparin sodium is an injectable anticoagulant that can be given intravenously or subcutaneously for more acute illnesses such as deep vein thrombosis, myocardial infarction, and pulmonary embolism. Partial thromboplastin time (PTT), PT, and INR will be monitored frequently. Heparin sodium is used cautiously in the patient who has/or will be undergoing surgery.

Hypertensive patients with heart failure

Optimal treatment goals for the hypertensive patient with heart failure is to reach a stable blood pressure of less than 130/80 mmHg. This usually requires more than one medication. An angiotensin-converting enzyme (ACE) inhibitor with thiazide diuretic therapy slows cardiac remodeling, improves cardiac function, and reduces further cardiovascular events after a myocardial infarction. Beta-blockers are also commonly added. Other medications that might be considered are dihydropyridine calcium antagonists, angiotensin receptor blockers (ARBs), aldosterone inhibitors, and isosorbide dinitrate/hydralazine.

Opioid rotation

Opioid rotation is a process of systematically switching a patient's prescribed opioid when they no longer seem to be receiving effective pain relief on their current medication, rather than increasing the dosage. Changing from one opioid to another, or altering the delivery method, may become necessary under the assumption that incomplete cross-tolerance among opioids occurs. Changing analgesics or the method of delivery may result in a decreased drug requirement. When altering opioid delivery regimes, use morphine equivalents as the common factor for all dose conversions. This method will help reduce medication errors.

Spasmolytics

Spasmolytics for the bladder include flavoxate hydrochloride (Urispas), oxybutynin chloride (Ditropan, Oxytrol), phenazopyridine hydrochloride (AZO-Standard, Geridium, Pyridium, Urodine), and tolterodine tartrate (Detrol). These are used to offer relief to patients with urinary disorders such as urinary frequency, urgency, nocturia, incontinence, pain, and bladder spasms.

Carisoprodol, cyclobenzaprine, metaxalone, and methocarbamol are used in conjunction with rest and physical therapy to treat acute/painful musculoskeletal conditions causing muscle spasms. These conditions frequently include fibromyalgia, tension headaches, and myofascial pain syndrome. These are contraindicated in neurological conditions such as cerebral palsy and multiple sclerosis.

Antiarrhythmic drugs

Advantages and disadvantages

Antiarrhythmic drugs include sodium-channel blockers, beta-blockers, potassium-channel blockers, calcium-channel blocker, adenosine, digitalis, atropine, and even electrolyte supplements when given for the express purpose of helping to correct a cardiac rhythm anomaly. It is important to understand the action of each medication and match it carefully to the individual patient's needs. Antiarrhythmics are always given with caution because they not only stabilize cardiac excitability or depression, but they could also cause a secondary arrhythmia or other unwanted cardiac complication such as hypotension.

Otitis media

The current recommendation by the American Academy of Pediatrics is a 10-day course of amoxicillin. Secondary choices are erythromycin or sulfonamide. It is important to note that some cases of otitis media are viral in origin and require no antibiotic. These ear infections will resolve on their own. Treatment with antibiotics may be delayed by 48 to 72 hours in the child between the ages of 6 months to 2 years to avoid overuse of antibiotics if the cause may be viral in origin.

ACE inhibitors

Angiotensin-converting enzyme (ACE) inhibitors are used to lower blood pressure by promoting vasodilation as well as acting as a diuretic. This is a recommended treatment option for heart failure patients and those recovering from myocardial infarction. ACE inhibitors are identified by the ending "pril": benazepril, captopril, enalapril, fosinopril, lisinopril, moexipril, quinapril, and ramipril. Side effects are rare, but the patient may experience some dizziness or lightheadedness when therapy begins. ACE inhibitors should not be taken during pregnancy or when breastfeeding.

Beta-blockers

Beta-blockers (β-blockers) block norepinephrine and epinephrine from binding with their receptors to slow the heartbeat and lower blood pressure. These include acebutolol, bisoprolol, esmolol, propranolol, atenolol, labetalol, carvedilol, and metoprolol. Note the identifying ending of "lol." β-blockers are recommended for the diabetic patient, cardiac arrhythmias, heart failure, myocardial infarction recovery, and angina pectoris. β-blockers are generally not used in combination with calcium-channel blockers. Side effects are rare, but β-blockers are able to cross the blood–brain barrier, and this may result in central nervous system (CNS) symptoms such as headache or dizziness. β-blockers may also mask symptoms of hypoglycemia and exacerbate asthma. Gradual tapering over one to two weeks is advisable. Abrupt cessation can lead to rebound hypertension, tachycardia, sweating, unstable angina, myocardial infarction, and possibly death.

Calcium-channel blockers

Calcium-channel blockers (amlodipine, felodipine, diltiazem, verapamil, nifedipine, nicardipine, nisoldipine, and bepridil) relax blood vessels and reduce cardiac workload by preventing calcium from entering the cardiac tissue. This lowers pulse and blood pressure. They may be prescribed for cardiac disease, coronary spasms or angina, arrhythmias, hypertrophic cardiomyopathy, or right-sided heart failure. Patients should be educated not to eat or drink grapefruit or consume alcohol while on this medication. Dosages may need to be lowered in older adults because they are more prone to side effects.

Parkinson's disease

A combination of levodopa and carbidopa (Sinemet, Parcopa) is the treatment of choice for Parkinson's disease. Levodopa acts to reduce tremor, rigidity, bradykinesia, and postural inability, but it cannot slow or halt disease progression. Carbidopa facilitates the ability of levodopa to reach the brain in optimal amounts. When it is working well, mobility is improved; however, the patient can experience dyskinesia. There is also a varied cycle of effectiveness with prolonged use. When the medication is less effective, motor symptoms become more spasmodic and unpredictable. Possible interactions may be experienced when the patient is also taking antacids, antiseizure medications, antihypertensives, antidepressants, and a high-protein consumption.

Impetigo

Impetigo is a common bacterial skin infection caused by streptococcus, staphylococcus, or methicillin-resistant *Staphylococcus aureus* (MRSA) that enters through a break in the skin. Impetigo appears as a single or multiple blisters filled with clear, yellow fluid that burst easily. These leave behind a red, raw area of irritation. The rash is most common on the face and lips but may spread to other areas. It is contagious. Mupirocin ointment is recommended for treatment, but oral antibiotics may be needed for severe cases.

Constipation

Before medication is considered, review the patient's fiber and fluid intake, as well as his or her activity level. Encourage dietary modifications, exercise, and bowel training activities before a prescription is issued. Medication choices fall into four categories, listed by order of choice: bulk laxatives, stool softeners, osmotic laxatives, and stimulant laxatives.

Bulk laxatives (methylcellulose, polycarbophil, and psyllium) are dietary fiber supplements taken when the patient's normal consumption is still inadequate.

Stool softeners, also called emollient laxatives, (docusate calcium, docusate sodium) encourage water to enter into the bowel.

Osmotic laxatives (lactulose, magnesium citrate, magnesium hydroxide, polyethylene glycol, sodium biphosphate, and sorbitol) stimulate osmosis and create more available water in the intestine.

Stimulant laxatives (bisacodyl, cascara sagrada, castor oil, and senna) encourage greater intestinal motility and increase water in the bowel.

Oral contraceptives

Hormone-based oral contraceptives are the most common choice among women for birth control. But this method is not recommended for women older than age 35 with a history of smoking, high blood pressure, or thrombosis. The most common types of oral contraceptives are often a combination of both estrogen and progestin; these are preferable and most effective when used with accuracy. Effectiveness may be altered by rifampin and antiepileptics, phenytoin, and carbamazepine. The patient must also be aware that oral contraceptives do not prevent the spread of HIV or STDs. Oral contraceptives may also be prescribed to stabilize symptoms of premenstrual syndrome (PMS) or help treat acne. Progesterone-only contraceptives are recommended for the breastfeeding patient.

Emergency contraception

Emergency contraception can be provided to women who have a fear that they may have been unintentionally impregnated. This may occur because of sexual assault or rape, protective device failure (condom breakage or dislodged diaphragm), or when no birth control was used at all (including forgetting to regularly take prescribed birth control pills). Two emergency contraceptive pills are available without a prescription: Plan B One-Step and Next Choice. Ulipristal requires a prescription. Any of these methods can be taken up to five days after the unprotected sex occurs.

Antipsychotics

First-generation antipsychotics include haloperidol, chlorpromazine, perphenazine, and fluphenazine. They are used to treat schizophrenia and related disorders. These antipsychotics can produce Parkinson-like symptoms such as akinesia, bradykinesia, stoic facial expression, tremor, cogwheel rigidity, postural abnormalities, and tardive dyskinesia.

Second-generation (atypical) antipsychotics include clozapine, risperidone, olanzapine, quetiapine, ziprasidone, aripiprazole and paliperidone. Special care must be taken when prescribing clozapine to monitor the patient's white blood cell count. Other medications should be considered before clozapine. Atypical antipsychotics often cause weight gain.

NSAIDs in rheumatoid arthritis

NSAIDs (naproxen) can be used to treat symptoms and pain related to diseases such as rheumatoid arthritis, but they cannot slow or halt disease progression. Patients may benefit from NSAID use through its anti-inflammatory, analgesic, and antipyretic properties. NSAIDs tend to be the first line of defense against pain caused by inflammatory conditions. They may also be used in conjunction with opioid therapy to reduce the amount of opioid needed. Adversely, gastrointestinal bleeding or ulceration, decreased renal function, and impaired platelet aggregation may occur. Studies have also indicated that the therapeutic effects of NSAIDs may not extend beyond six to twelve months of use. Short-term memory loss may occur in older patients. There may be an increased cardiovascular risk with prolonged use. Patients allergic to sulfa drugs can also experience a cross-sensitivity to some types of NSAIDs.

Triptans

Triptans (sumatriptan, eletriptan, almotriptan, frovatriptan, rizatriptan, zolmitriptan) are serotonin receptor agonists that help relieve pain from acute migraine attacks by causing vasoconstriction of the intracranial blood vessels and relieving swelling. Sensitivity to light and noise, nausea and vomiting also associated with migraines will be quickly resolved as well. Combining triptans with acetaminophen or naproxen can boost its effectiveness even further. They can cause irritation at the point of administration (injection or nasal spray) and may cause some dizziness, drowsiness, or lightheadedness. Triptans cannot be used in patients with cerebrovascular disease. Patients should also be educated about rebound headaches.

Metronidazole

Oral metronidazole (Flagyl) is an antibiotic used to treat infections of the reproductive system or gastrointestinal tract such as pelvic inflammatory disease (PID), trichomoniasis, and *Clostridium difficile* (C-diff). Nausea and headache are common side effects. Flagyl may also be given intravenously.

Topical cream metronidazole is applied to the skin once a day for the treatment of rosacea. It does not, however, cure the disease process. It may also be used as vaginal treatment for bacterial infections (two times a day for five days). Either application has the potential to cause skin irritation.

Adverse side effects versus an allergic reaction to a medication

Nonallergic reaction: Although adverse side effects can be, at times, very severe, the body does not form antibodies against the medication.

Allergic reaction: A true allergic reaction means that the body's immune system has created antibodies against the foreign substance it perceives as a threat. These antibodies cause an anaphylaxis reaction with hives, facial and throat swelling, wheezing, light-headedness, vomiting, and even shock. These reactions are almost immediate, occurring in under an hour, although there may be a delay of several hours.

Permethrin cream

Over-the-counter permethrin 1% cream can be used to treat lice. Permethrin 5% (Elimite) cream can be prescribed as treatment for scabies. The patient should be instructed to wash and dry their entire body, then apply the cream to every exposed surface, paying particular attention to the creases and folds. Permethrin 5% cream needs to remain on the skin for at least 8 to 14 hours. Then the patient should again wash and dry thoroughly and put on clean clothing. Patients should be aware that the itching will ease somewhat within the first 24 hours but may not be completely relieved for up to 4 weeks after treatment. It may also cause temporary redness of the skin as well. Permethrin is safe for use in infants after 2 months of age through the elderly.

Obesity

Most common health risks

Obesity is defined as a body mass index (BMI) of 30 or greater. Children and adults who are obese are at a greater risk for developing gallstones, diabetes, high blood pressure, high cholesterol and triglyceride levels, coronary artery disease, stroke, and sleep apnea. If the distribution of fat is more toward a lower, pear-shaped body frame, it carries a slightly lower risk than those who carry a more central, stomach-fat distribution. Likewise, those who are able to lose weight and maintain a healthy lifestyle can reduce the chance of these health risks.

Panic attacks

Long-term treatment and prevention of panic attacks can often be treated by antidepressants. Selective serotonin reuptake inhibitors (SSRIs) such as fluoxetine (Prozac), paroxetine (Paxil), citalopram (Celexa), escitalopram (Lexapro), and sertraline (Zoloft) are the initial choices. The next choice is selective serotonin and norepinephrine reuptake inhibitors (SSNRIs). Treatment of an acute attack requires a sedative such as Xanax, Klonopin, Valium, or Ativan.

In addition to medication, psychotherapy, cognitive-behavioral therapy, relaxation, and meditation training should also be considered.

Upper respiratory infections

Upper respiratory infections are the most common cause of doctor visits. An upper respiratory infection involves the sinuses, nasal passages, pharynx, and larynx. There is typically inflammation of these areas that causes pain, congestion, and cough. The patient may also complain of difficulty breathing and fatigue. These types of illnesses are most common during the fall and winter months. The virus is contagious through respiratory droplets that are inhaled or transferred by touch. The risk of contracting an upper respiratory infection is highest among those who spend long hours in close quarters with many other people, those with poor hand-washing habits, smokers, immunocompromised individuals, and those working in health-care settings. It is not caused by a bacterial infection and cannot be relieved through the use of antibiotics.

ADHD

Attention-deficit hyperactivity disorder (ADHD) must be properly diagnosed in order for prescribed medications to have the desired effect. The most common classification of medication used is psychostimulants: amphetamine-dextroamphetamine (Adderall), dexmethylphenidate (Focalin), dextroamphetamine (Dexedrine), lisdexamfetamine (Vyvanse), and methylphenidate (Ritalin). In true ADHD, these drugs have a calming effect on the patient rather than a stimulating effect. The nonstimulant atomoxetine (Strattera) may also be considered. The first line of choice for treatment in a newly diagnosed younger child is behavioral therapy. Medication should be prescribed only after prudent consideration and continued close patient contact to monitor its effects.

Gentamicin

Gentamicin is an antibiotic used to treat bacterial infections. In its injectable form, it is often used to treat serious infections such as *Pseudomonas, Escherichia coli,* and *Staphylococcus*. Standard dosing is 1 mg/kg every 8 hours. Common side effects include nausea, vomiting, and loss of appetite. When given as an intramuscular injection, patients often complain of pain and irritation at the injection site. Gentamicin in this form also carries a high risk of renal and ototoxicity.

Gentamicin can also be prescribed in a solution for use as eyedrops to treat infections such as conjunctivitis.

Interventions for back pain

Depending on the source, amount, and consistency of the pain, treatment options can vary greatly. Treatment options include: physical therapy, mild anti-inflammatory medications, chiropractic referrals, transcutaneous electrical nerve stimulation (TENS) or intradiscal electrothermal therapy (IDET) units, injections, and surgical interventions. Any intervention is aimed at reducing pain and recovering movement. For an acute episode, an ice pack and anti-inflammatory agent may be sufficient. Long-term bed rest is not recommended. For more chronic needs, treatment options should progress from the most noninvasive that is needed for the patient to receive relief.

Doxorubicin

Doxorubicin is an antineoplastic drug common in the treatment of breast, bladder, ovarian, and endometrial cancers. It may also be used in certain types of lymphoma and leukemia, thyroid, and skin cancers. Injections are provided every 21 to 28 days. Common side effects include nausea, vomiting, mouth and throat lesions, changes in appetite, fatigue, and weight loss. Long-term monitoring of the heart should also be planned for because doxorubicin can have a damaging effect on cardiac health.

Salicylic acid

Salicylic acid is a popular medication used for treatment of various skin disorders such as psoriasis, ichthyoses, dandruff, corns, calluses, and warts. It works by reducing swelling, redness, and irritation while unclogging pores in the treatment of acne. For other conditions, it loosens and softens areas of thickened or calloused skin until it falls off naturally or can be easily removed. Mild concentrations are used for most conditions. Solutions of 2% to 10% concentration are used for treatment of corns and up to 17% for warts. However, salicylic acid should not be used to treat warts on the face, mouth or nose; any wart with a hair follicle; genital warts; moles; or birthmarks.

Antihistamines

Antihistamines are chemically designed to block histamines that are triggered by allergies in order to calm the body's reaction to the invasive organism. Not every antihistamine works for every symptom that may be experienced. The most marked side effect of first-generation antihistamines (diphenhydramine, clemastine) is a greater risk of sedation than second-generation antihistamines (loratadine, fexofenadine, desloratadine). All of these medications can also cause patient complaints of dry mouth and mucous membranes, dizziness, restlessness or change in mood, and occasionally nausea and vomiting.

Types of insulin

Rapid-acting insulin (Humalog, NovoLog, Apidra) is designed to act on the body's needs for insulin during meal consumption. Its peak is within 30 minutes to 1 ½ hours, and its full duration of action is between 1 to 5 hours.

Short-acting insulin (regular Humulin, Velosulin) is used when a meal is anticipated within 30 minutes to an hour. Peak action is 2 to 5 hours, and the duration is 2 to 8 hours.

Intermediate-acting insulin (NPH, Lente) covers an extended period such as the time when the patient is asleep, and their need will be steady. Peak action is anywhere from 3 to 12 hours, and the full duration is 18 to 24 hours.

Long-acting insulin (Ultralente, Lantus, Levemir) gives coverage for a full 24 hours. Peaks are very gentle or nonexistent, and the duration is 24 to 36 hours.

Premixed: Combinations of insulin with different durations can be premixed to provide a more complex level of coverage. Premixed insulins include Humulin 70/30, Novolin 70/30, NovoLog 70/30, Humulin 50/50, and Humalog mix 75/25.

Addiction and pseudoaddiction

Addiction is a primary and constant neurobiologic disease with genetic, psychosocial, and environmental factors that create an obsessive and irrational need or preoccupation with a substance. Addictive behaviors include unrestricted, continued cravings, and compulsive and persistent use of a drug despite harmful experiences and side effect.

Pseudoaddiction is an assumption that the patient is addicted to a substance, when in actuality the patient is not experiencing relief from the medication. It is prolonged, unrelieved pain that may be the result of undertreatment. This situation may lead the patient to become more aggressive in seeking medicated relief, thus resulting in the inappropriate "drug-seeker" label.

Physical dependence, tolerance, and pseudotolerance

Physical dependence is a condition of bodily adaptation to the presence of a specific drug or chemical. Abrupt removal or a rapid reduction of dosage will result in withdrawal symptoms. The patient does not present with the psychological and environmental dependence that are evident in addictions, such as an obsessive and irrational need or preoccupation with a substance, unrestricted, continued cravings, and compulsive and persistent use of a drug despite harmful experiences and side effects.

Tolerance is the adaptation of the body to continued exposure to a drug or chemical. The effects of the drug at the same level of exposure are minimized over time. Additional dosing is required to maintain the same outcomes.

Pseudotolerance is the misguided perception of the caregiver that a patient's need for increasing doses of a drug is due to the development of tolerance, when in reality disease progression or other factors are responsible for the increase in dosing needs.

Applying Basic Science Concepts

Parameters for dystocia

Dystocia is defined as an abnormal or difficult childbirth. This is a condition that occurs in approximately 20% of pregnancies. Complications can range from uncoordinated uterine contractions, abnormal fetal presentation, or cephalopelvic disproportion. The form of dystocia most often referred to is shoulder dystocia, in which the infant's shoulder presents into the birth canal first, making it impossible for the labor and delivery to progress naturally. Those women whose pregnancies occur too close together or too far apart, primigravida, and multiparous pregnancies are most often affected.

G6PD deficiency

Glucose-6-phosphate dehydrogenase deficiency (G6PD) is a genetic disorder in which the red blood cells undergo hemolysis. This disease process causes hemolytic anemia. The patient may present with pale skin, jaundice, dark urine, complaints of extreme fatigue, difficulty breathing, and an increased heart rate. This condition is not constant. Many people will not ever experience symptoms and complications from the disorder. Hemolysis may result from infection, medication, or allergen triggers (most often fava bean). G6PD is more common in males than females.

Normal heart sounds

Heart sounds are actually created by the noise of the blood pushing through the heart valves. S1, or the "lub" sound, is created by the mitral and tricuspid valves. S2, or the "dub" sound, is created by the aortic and pulmonary valves.

During youth, a third benign heart sound, S3, or gallop, may also be present after S2. In the adult, this is an indication of cardiac disease.

Abnormal sounds that might be observed occur when these valves do not close at the proper times or do not close completely.

Abnormal breathing patterns

Cheyne-Stokes: respiratory depression caused by heart failure and uremia.

Kussmaul: deep, rapid, labored breathing related to acidosis.

Obstructive: obstructive lung disease, or COPD, causing prolonged expiration due to narrowed airways and increased resistance.

Ataxic: unpredictable irregularity, both shallow and deep breaths, apnea, from brain damage and respiratory depression.

Tachypnea: rapid shallow breathing, with multiple causes.

Hypovolemia

Hypovolemia is a state of decreased blood plasma volume. Common causes of hypovolemia are dehydration, bleeding, vomiting, and burns. Dehydration can be a cause, but is not interchangeable with the term hypovolemia. Dehydration is a decrease in the available water within the body. A specific loss of blood plasma (hypovolemia) also includes a marked depletion in sodium levels as well. If the loss is greater than 10% to 20% of the body's total volume, the patient can begin to exhibit symptoms such as tachycardia, hypotension, pale skin, dizziness, change in mental status, nausea, and excessive thirst. Hypovolemia shock can also result. If needed, treatment involves both fluid and blood plasma replacement.

Frank-Starling law of the heart

Frank–Starling law (also known as Starling's law or Maestrini heart's law) describes the correlation between cardiac blood volume and stroke volume. End diastolic volume is directly proportional to stroke volume. The greater the amount of fluid within the ventricles during diastole, the greater the amount of force that will be exerted during the systolic contraction. This process is independent from any neural or hormonal influences. When the heart's ability to contract is compromised, heart failure may be suspect. The heart will resort to the law of Laplace to try and compensate, and S3 may be detected.

law of Laplace

The Frank–Starling law describes the correlation between cardiac blood volume and stroke volume. End diastolic volume is directly proportional to stroke volume. The greater the amount of fluid within the ventricles during diastole, the greater the amount of force will be exerted during the systolic contraction. If there is a reduced surface tension and the amount of blood being circulated becomes unstable, amphipathic phospholipid-based pulmonary surfactant allows alveoli to remain open in an attempt to increase the oxygenation to the circulating blood volume. If this process remains unchecked, an aneurysm can result.

Poiseuille's law/equation

Poiseuille's law explains the relationship between pressure and resistance that affects blood or air flow. The longer the length and smaller the size of a lumen creates greater resistance, making an increased pressure need that raises blood pressure and decreases oxygenation. The equation is as follows: (volume flow rate) is equal to (pi divided by eight) times (the pressure difference between the ends of the tube) times (the radius of the tube to the fourth power) divided by (the viscosity, or thickness, of the fluid) divided by (the length of the tube).

Sodium-glucose transport proteins

Sodium glucose linked transporters (SGLTs) are found in the mucous membranes of the small intestines. Their role is to help with renal glucose reabsorption because sodium and glucose transport across membranes in the same direction. In cases where blood glucose levels have become too high, SGLT allows glucose to be excreted in the urine by creating a sodium gradient for the glucose to follow. This knowledge is currently being explored for its usefulness in treating type 2 diabetes mellitus.

Purine metabolism

Purine and xanthine are nucleotides involved in both DNA and RNA formation as well as energy transference and nitrogen disposal. The purine family includes adenine, guanine, caffeine, xanthine, uric acid, and others. Purine is metabolized by hypoxanthine-guanine phosphoribosyltransferase (HPRT). Disruptions in this process can cause DNA genetic disorders that are hereditary. Health problems such as Lesch–Nyhan syndrome, gout, anemia, epilepsy, developmental delays, deafness, kidney disease, and immune disorders as well as many others can be caused by the resulting disruptions in the purine metabolism that in turn cause DNA disruptions. The action of allopurinol inhibits the conversion of xanthine into uric acid, making it an effective treatment for gout.

Function of the sinoatrial (SA) node

The cells of the sinoatrial (SA) node are specialized to act automatically, regardless of the electrical impulses in the surrounding cardiac tissue. This allows it to act as the pacemaker for the heart. The impulses travel from the SA node to the atrioventricular (AV) node, through it to the bundle of His and Perkinje fibers to the rest of the cardiac tissues causing coordinated contractions. The SA node's natural rhythm is a steady 60 to 70 beats per minute. If there is a greater oxygen demand by the cells of the body, this message is relayed to the SA node, which responds by sending out more rapid impulses to increase blood circulation through the heart and lungs to the body. If there is a malfunction of the SA node, the AV node will act as a fail-safe and take over the regulation of the heart at a slightly slower rhythm.

Cause and risks of condyloma acuminata

Condyloma acuminata (genital warts) are caused by a contact infection with any one of more than 100 types of human papillomavirus (HPV). The most common types are types 6 and 11. The risk is highest between the ages of 17 and 33 among those who begin sexual activity at an early age, smoke, use oral contraceptives, have a previous history of a sexually transmitted disease (STD), have a compromised immune system, and have multiple sexual partners of both sexes. It may be difficult to pinpoint the origin of the infection if multiple partners are involved because the initial stages have no discernible symptoms. Lesions generally develop up to three months after contact. Identification of genital warts during pregnancy is important because the virus can also be passed to the infant during birth. Genital warts also increase the patient's risk for later developing cancer.

Effects of the AIDS virus on the patient's cells

The AIDS virus attaches itself to the CD4 cell surface protein of T-4 lymphocytes with a viral envelope of glycoprotein (gp120). This protein binds to CD4 receptors and coreceptors (CXCR4 and CCR5). HIV is a retrovirus that quickly infects circulating immune cells or finds safe harbors in body reservoirs that are inaccessible to drug therapy. The retrovirus uses an enzyme called reverse transcriptase to convert the HIV viral RNA to a viral DNA. This conversion allows the viral DNA to take over the host cell DNA of lymphocytes, macrophages, and other immune system cells. When the viral DNA has taken over, it produces viral proteins that assemble into virions using viral enzyme protease. Each reproductive cycle of HIV can produce up to 100 billion virions with minor protective mutations. The CD4 count indicates disease severity. Less than 500 cells/mm^3 is found in the early symptomatic stage. A count less than 200 and a viral load greater than 100,000/ml are found in the late symptomatic stage.

Practice Test

Practice Questions

Note: The length of the review material in this document indicates the broad scope of the PANCE Test content. These questions provide 4 answer choices for each question. On the actual exam there may be more than 4 answer choices on some questions.

1. A P.A. is working in an outpatient orthopedic clinic. During the patient's history the patient reports, "I tore 3 of my 4 Rotator cuff muscles in the past." Which of the following muscles cannot be considered as possibly being torn?
   a. Teres minor
   b. Teres major
   c. Supraspinatus
   d. Infraspinatus

2. A P.A. at an outpatient clinic is determining the appropriate sequence to arrange patients in the afternoon. Which of the following calls should have the highest priority for medical intervention?
   a. A home health patient reports, "I am starting to have breakdown of my heels."
   b. A patient that received an upper extremity cast yesterday reports, "I can't feel my fingers in my right hand today."
   c. A young female reports, "I think I sprained my ankle about 2 weeks ago."
   d. A middle-aged patient reports, "My knee is still hurting from the TKR."

3. A P.A. working a surgical unit notices a patient is experiencing SOB, calf pain, and warmth over the posterior calf. All of these may indicate which of the following medical conditions?
   a. Patient may have a DVT.
   b. Patient may be exhibiting signs of dermatitis.
   c. Patient may be in the late phases of CHF.
   d. Patient may be experiencing anxiety after surgery.

4. A P.A. is performing a screening on a patient that has been casted recently on the left lower extremity. Which of the following statements should the P.A. be most concerned about?
   a. The patient reports, "I didn't keep my extremity elevated like the P.A. asked me to."
   b. The patient reports, "I have been having pain in my left calf."
   c. The patient reports, "My left leg has really been itching."
   d. The patient reports "The arthritis in my wrists is flaring up, when I put weight on my crutches."

5. The bacteria *Neisseria gonorrhoeae* can be classified as a:
   a. Gram-negative cocci
   b. Spirochetes
   c. Acid-fast bacilli
   d. Gram-positive cocci

6. The bacteria *Staphylococcus aureus* can be classified as a:
   a. Gram-negative cocci
   b. Spirochetes
   c. Acid-fast bacilli
   d. Gram-positive cocci

7. A P.A. has just started on the 7PM surgical shift rotation. Which of the following patients should the P.A. check on first?
   a. A 75 year-old female who is scheduled for an EGD in 10 hours.
   b. A 34 year-old male who is complaining of low back pain following back surgery and has an onset of urinary incontinence in the last hour.
   c. A 21 year-old male who had a lower extremity BKA yesterday, following a MVA and has phantom pain.
   d. A 27 year-old female who has received 1.5 units of RBC's. via transfusion the previous day.

8. A 22 year-old patient in a mental health lock-down unit under suicide watch appears happy about being discharged. Which of the following is probably happening?
   a. The patient is excited about being around family again.
   b. The patient's suicide plan has probably progressed.
   c. The patient's plans for the future have been clarified.
   d. The patient's mood is improving.

9. Which of the following microorganisms has not been linked to Meningitis?
   a. Flavobacterium meningosepticum
   b. Listeria monocytogenes
   c. Pasteurella multocida
   d. *Streptobacillus moniliformis*

10. A 13 year old girl is admitted to the hospital with lower right abdominal discomfort. The P.A. should take which the following measures first?
   a. Administer Loritab to the patient for pain relief.
   b. Place the patient in right sidelying position for pressure relief.
   c. Start a Central Line.
   d. Provide pain reduction techniques without administering medication.

11. A patient that has TB can be taken off restrictions after which of the following parameters have been met?
   a. Negative culture results.
   b. After 30 days of isolation.
   c. Normal body temperature for 48 hours.
   d. Non-productive cough for 72 hours.

12. A P.A. teaching a patient with COPD pulmonary exercises should do which of the following?
   a. Teach purse-lip breathing techniques.
   b. Encourage repetitive heavy lifting exercises that will increase strength.
   c. Limit exercises based on respiratory acidosis.
   d. Take breaks every 10-20 minutes with exercises.

13. A patient asks a P.A. the following question. Exposure to TB can be identified best with which of the following procedures?

a. Chest x-ray
b. Mantoux test
c. Breath sounds examination
d. Sputum culture for gram-negative bacteria

14. A fifty-five year-old man suffered a left frontal lobe CVA. The patient's family is not present in the room. Which of the following should the P.A. watch most closely for?

a. Changes in emotion and behavior
b. Monitor loss of hearing
c. Observe appetite and vision deficits
d. Changes in facial muscle control

15. A central venous pressure reading of 11cm/H(2)0 of an IV of normal saline is determined by the P.A. caring for the patient. The patient has a diagnosis of pericarditis. Which of the following is the most applicable:

a. The patient has a condition of hypovolemia.
b. Not enough fluid has been given to the patient.
c. Pericarditis may cause pressures greater than 10cm/H(2)0 with testing of CVP.
d. The patient may have a condition of arteriosclerosis.

16. A physician is instructing a patient on the order of sensations with the application of an ice water bath for a swollen right ankle. Which of the following is the correct order of sensations experienced with an ice water bath?

a. cold, burning, aching, and numbness
b. burning, aching, cold, and numbness
c. aching, cold, burning and numbness
d. cold, aching, burning and numbness

17. A P.A. consults with a male patient that has a diagnosis of CAD and COPD. The patient is currently taking Ventolin, Azmacort, Aspirin, and Theophylline. The patient complains of upset stomach, nausea and feeling uncomfortable. The P.A. should:

a. Monitor the patient for theophylline toxicity.
b. Recommend the patient position himself in right sidelying.
c. Recommend the patient schedule a P.A.'s visit in one week.
d. Recommend a hold on the drug-Azmacort

18. A P.A. reviewed the arterial blood gas reading of a 25 year-old male. The P.A. should be able to conclude the patient is experiencing which of the following conditions?

Bicarbonate Ion-25 mEq/l	*PaO2-54 mmHg*
PH-7.41	*(FiO2)-.22*
PaCO2-29 mmHg	

a. metabolic acidosis
b. respiratory acidosis
c. metabolic alkalosis
d. respiratory alkalosis

19. Syphilis has been directly linked to?
    a. Streptococcus (anaerobic species)
    b. Treponema pallidum
    c. Borrelia burgdorferi
    d. Chlamydia *trachomatis*

20. Tricyclics (Antidepressants) sometimes have which of the following adverse affects on patients that have a diagnosis of depression?
    a. Shortness of breath
    b. Fainting
    c. Large Intestine ulcers
    d. Distal muscular weakness

21. A P.A. is instructing a patient about the warning signs of (Digitalis) side effects. Which of the following side effects should the P.A. tell the patient are sometimes associated with excessive levels of Digitalis?
    a. Seizures
    b. Muscle weakness
    c. Depression
    d. Anxiety

22. A P.A. is assessing a patient's right lower extremity. The extremity is warm to touch, red and swollen. The patient is also running a low fever. Which of the following conditions would be the most likely cause of the patient's condition?
    a. Herpes
    b. Scleroderma
    c. Dermatitis
    d. Cellulitis

23. A P.A. is assessing a patient's breath sounds. The patient has had a pneumonectomy to the right lung performed 48 hours ago. Which of the following conditions most likely exists?
    a. Decreased breath sound volume
    b. Elevated tidal volume
    c. Elevated respiratory capacity
    d. Wheezing

24. A P.A. is assessing a patient in the ICU. The patient has the following signs: weak pulse, quick respiration, acetone breath, and nausea. Which of the following conditions is most likely occurring?
    a. Hypoglycemic patient
    b. Hyperglycemic patient
    c. Cardiac arrest
    d. End-stage renal failure

25. Medical records indicate a patient has developed a condition of respiratory alkalosis. Which of the following clinical signs would not apply to a condition of respiratory alkalosis?
    a. Muscle tetany
    b. Syncope
    c. Numbness
    d. Anxiety

26. Which of the following lab values would indicate symptomatic AIDS in the medical chart? (T4 cell count per deciliter)

a. Greater than 1000 cells per deciliter
b. Less than 500 cells per deciliter
c. Greater than 2000 cells per deciliter
d. Less than 200 cells per deciliter

27. A P.A. is assessing a 18 year-old female who has recently suffered a TBI. The P.A. notes a slower pulse and impaired respiration. The patient is experiencing which of the following conditions?

a. Increased intracranial pressure
b. Increased function of cranial nerve X
c. Sympathetic response to activity
d. Meningitis

28. A P.A. taking a patient's history realizes the patient is complaining of SOB and weakness in the lower extremities. The patient has a history of hyperlipidemia, and hypertension. Which of the following may be occurring?

a. The patient is developing CHF
b. The patient may be having a MI
c. The patient may be developing COPD
d. The patient may be having an onset of PVD

29. A P.A. has been assigned a patient who has recently been diagnosed with Guillain-Barre' Syndrome. Which of the following statements is the most applicable when discussing the impairments with Guillain-Barre' Syndrome with the patient?

a. Guillain-Barre' Syndrome gets better after 5 years in almost all cases.
b. Guillain-Barre' Syndrome causes limited sensation in the abdominal region.
c. Guillain-Barre' Syndrome causes muscle weakness in the legs.
d. Guillain-Barre' Syndrome does not affect breathing in severe cases.

30. Which of the following is not considered a RNA related virus?

a. Cytomegalovirus
b. Rabies virus
c. Influenza virus
d. Poliovirus

31. A P.A. is assessing a patient in the rehab unit. The patient has suffered a TBI 3 weeks ago. Which of the following is the most distinguishing characteristic of a neurological disturbance?

a. LOC (level of consciousness)
b. Short term memory
c. + Babinski sign
d. + Clonus sign

32. Which of the following microorganisms has not been linked directly to UTI's?

a. Proteus mirabilis
b. Streptococcus faecalis
c. Escherichia coli
d. Streptococcus *pneumoniae*

33. A P.A. is caring for a patient in the step down unit. The patient has signs of increased intracranial pressure. Which of the following is not a sign of increased intracranial pressure?
a. Bradycardia
b. Increased pupil size bilaterally
c. Change in LOC
d. Vomiting

34. The charge nurse on a cardiac unit tells you a patient is exhibiting signs of right-sided heart failure. Which of the following would not indicate right-sided heart failure?
a. Nausea
b. Anorexia
c. Rapid weight gain
d. SOB (shortness of breath)

35. A 62 year-old female is being seen at an outpatient clinic by a P.A. The patient reports she has been taking Premarin for years to the P.A. Which of the following would indicate an over-dosage of Premarin in this case?
a. Lower extremity edema
b. Sensory changes in the upper extremities
c. Increased occurrence of fractures
d. Decreased peripheral blood flow

36. A 46 year-old has returned from a heart catheterization and wants to get up to start walking 3 hours after the procedure. The P.A. should:
a. Tell the patient to remain with the leg straight for at least another hour.
b. Allow the patient to begin limited ambulation with assistance.
c. Ordera physical therapy consultation for ambulation.
d. Tell the patient to remain with leg straight for another 6 hours.

37. A P.A. is reviewing a patient's ECG report. The patient exhibits a flat T wave, depressed ST segment and short QT interval. Which of the following medications can cause all of the above effects?
a. Morphine
b. Atropine
c. Procardia
d. Digitalis

38. A patient has just been prescribed Minipress to control hypertension by a doctor. The P.A. should instruct the patient to be observant of the following:
a. Dizziness and light headed sensations
b. Weight gain
c. Sensory changes in the lower extremities
d. Fatigue

39. A patient is complaining of severe chest pain during a stress test. Which of the following medications is the most appropriate to relieve this discomfort?
a. Aspirin
b. Diazoxide
c. Procardia
d. Mannitol

40. A 15 year-old high school wrestler has been taking diuretics to lose weight to compete in a lower weight class. Which of the following medical tests is most like to be given?

a. Lab values of Potassium and Sodium
b. Lab values of glucose and hemoglobin
c. ECG
d. CT scan

41. A 55 year-old female asks a P.A. the following, "Which mineral/vitamin is the most important to prevent progression of osteoporosis. The P.A. should state:

a. Potassium
b. Magnesium
c. Calcium
d. Vitamin B12

42. A patient has recently been diagnosed with symptomatic bradycardia. Which of the following medications is the most recognized for treatment of symptomatic bradycardia?

a. Questran
b. Digitalis
c. Nitroglycerin
d. Atropine

43. A patient has recently been prescribed Lidocaine Hydrochloride. Which of the following symptoms may occur with over dosage?

a. Memory loss and lack of appetite
b. Confusion and fatigue
c. Heightened reflexes
d. Tinnitus and spasticity

44. A patient has recently been prescribed Albuterol. Which of the following changes are not associated with Albuterol?

a. Tachycardia
b. Hypertension
c. Bronchodilation
d. Sensory changes

45. Which of the following arterial blood gas values indicates a patient may be experiencing a condition of metabolic acidosis?

a. Pa02 (90%)
b. Bicarbonate 15.9 mmol/L
c. CO(2) 47 mm Hg
d. pH 7.34

46. A patient presents with a lesion in the brain with the following signs and symptoms: III cranical nerve involvement, ptosis, and contralateral hemiparesis. What is the location of the lesion?

a. Third ventricle
b. Midbrain
c. Pons
d. Precentral gyrus

47. A P.A. suspects a patient is developing Bell's Palsy. The P.A. wants to test the function of cranial nerve VII. Which of the following would be the most appropriate testing procedures?
a. Test the taste sensation over the back of the tongue and activation of the facial muscles.
b. Test the taste sensation over the front of the tongue and activation of the facial muscles.
c. Test the sensation of the facial muscles and sensation of the back of the tongue.
d. Test the sensation of the facial muscles and sensation of the front of the tongue.

48. A P.A. is reviewing a patient's serum glucose levels. Which of the following scenarios would indicate abnormal serum glucose values for a 30 year-old male.
a. 70 mg/dl
b. 55 mg/dl
c. 110 mg/dl
d. 100 mg/dl

49. A patient presents with a lesion in the brain with the following signs and symptoms: Contralateral hemiplegia, hemisensory loss and homonymous hemianopsia. What is the location of the lesion?
a. Internal capsule
b. Pineal gland
c. Prefrontal area
d. Uncus

50. A patient has recently been prescribed Zidovudine (Retrovir). The patient has AIDS. Which of the following side effects should the patient specifically watch out for?
a. Weakness and SOB
b. Fever and anemia
c. Hypertension and SOB
d. Fever and hypertension

51. A patient has recently been prescribed (Norvasc). Which of the following side effect/s should the patient specifically watch out for?
a. Hypotension and Angina
b. Hypertension
c. Lower extremity edema
d. Peripheral sensory loss and SOB

52. A P.A. is reviewing a patient's arterial blood gas values. Which of the following conditions apply under the following values?

pH- 7.49 *Pa02 – 52 mmHg*
Bicarbonate ion 24 mEq/dl *Fi02 - .22*
PaC02 – 31 mmHg

a. respiratory acidosis
b. respiratory alkalosis
c. metabolic acidosis
d. metabolic alkalosis

53. A 28 year-old male has a diagnosis of AIDS. The patient has had a two-year history of AIDS. The most like cognitive deficits include which of the following?
a. Disorientation
b. Sensory changes
c. Inability to produce sound
d. Hearing deficits

54. A patient has been admitted to the hospital with a HNP L4-5 segment diagnosis. After 24 hours the patient is able to ambulate with assistance with reduced muscle spasms. Which of the following medications was the most beneficial in changing the patient's mobility status?
a. Mivacron
b. Atropine
c. Bethanechol
d. Flexeril

55. Which of the following medications is not considered a neuromuscular blocker?
a. Anectine
b. Pavulon
c. Pitressin
d. Mivacron

56. A P.A. is caring for a 10 year-old boy who has just been diagnosed with a congenital heart defect. Which of the following clinical signs does not indicate congenital heart defect?
a. Increased body weight
b. Elevated heart rate
c. Lower extremity edema
d. Compulsive behavior

57. A patient presents with a lesion in the brain with the following signs and symptoms: Cranial nerve VI involvement, ipsilateral facial paralyis, locked-in syndrome, contralateral hemiparesis. What is the location of the lesion?
a. Internal capsule
b. Pons
c. Corpus callosum
d. Third ventricle

58. Which of the following effects is unrelated to Morphine's effects on a patient?
a. Depressed function of the CNS
b. Increased blood flow
c. Decreased venous capacity
d. Pain relief

59. A P.A. is reviewing a patient's current Lithium levels. Which of the following values is outside the therapeutic range?
a. 1.0 mEq/L
b. 1.1 mEq/L
c. 1.2 mEq/L
d. 1.3 mEq/L

60. Dermatome screening indicates sensory loss over the lateral forearm. Myotome screening indicates weak wrist extension on the same side. Which cervical nerve root level could be involved?
a. C4
b. C5
c. C6
d. C7

61. Which of the following side effects is not associated with Tegretol?
a. Sore throat
b. Vertigo
c. Fever
d. Shortness of breath

62. A doctor has prescribed Klonapin for the first time to a patient and asks the P.A., which of the following side effects is not associated with Klonapin?
a. Drowsiness
b. Ataxia
c. Salivation elevated
d. Diplopia

63. A patient has been diagnosed with diabetes mellitus. Which of the following is not a clinical sign of diabetes mellitus?
a. Polyphagia
b. Polyuria
c. Metabolic acidosis
d. Lower extremity edema

64. A patient has fallen off a bicycle and fractured the head of the proximal fibula. A cast was placed on the patient's lower extremity. Which of the following is the most probable result of the fall?
a. Peroneal nerve injury
b. Tibial nerve injury
c. Sciatic nerve injury
d. Femoral nerve injury

65. Which of the following applies to Buck's traction?
a. A weight greater than 10 lbs. should be used.
b. The line of pull is upward at an angle.
c. The line of pull is straight
d. A weight greater than 20 lbs. should be used.

66. Which of the following motions is identified with the corresponding action?
(Action- Turning palm of hand over to face in the anterior direction, dorsum of the hand is pointed downward toward the floor.)
a. Pronation
b. Supination
c. Abduction
d. Adduction

67. What type of cells secretes insulin?
   a. alpha cells
   b. beta cells
   c. CD4 cells
   d. helper cells

68. Which of the following is not considered one of the main mechanisms of Type II Diabetes treatment?
   a. Medications
   b. Nutrition
   c. Increased activity
   d. Continuous Insulin

69. What type of cells create exocrine secretions?
   a. alpha cells
   b. beta cells
   c. acinar cells
   d. plasma cells

70. A P.A. is caring for a patient who has experienced burns to the right lower extremity. According to the Rule of Nines which of the following percents most accurately describes the severity of the injury?
   a. 36%
   b. 27%
   c. 18%
   d. 9%

71. A patient has experienced a severe third degree burn to the trunk in the last 36 hours. Which phase of burn management is the patient in?
   a. Shock phase
   b. Emergent phase
   c. Healing phase
   d. Wound proliferation phase

72. A P.A. is reviewing a patient's medical record. The record indicates the patient has limited shoulder flexion on the left. Which plane of movement is limited?
   a. Horizontal
   b. Sagittal
   c. Frontal
   d. Vertical

73. What is the name of a tumor that tends to be encapsulated and is usually benign?
   a. Neuroma
   b. Meningioma
   c. Glioblastoma
   d. Lymphoma

74. If your patient is acutely psychotic, which of the following independent medical interventions would not be appropriate?

a. Conveying calmness with one on one interaction
b. Recognizing and dealing with your own feelings to prevent escalation of the patient's anxiety level
c. Encourage client participation in group therapy
d. Listen and identify causes of their behavior

75. A P.A. is teaching a client about self-administration of Haldol 15 mg po hs. For which side effect/s must the client seek medical attention?

a. SOB and fatigue
b. restlessness and muscle spasms
c. dry mouth
d. diarrhea

Answers and Explanations

1. B: Teres Minor, Infraspinatus, Supraspinatus, and Subscapularis make up the Rotator Cuff.

2. B: The patient experiencing neurovascular changes should have the highest priority. Pain following a TKR is normal, and breakdown over the heels is a gradual process. Moreover, a subacute ankle sprain is almost never a medical emergency.

3. A: All of these factors indicate a DVT.

4. B: Pain may be indicating neurovascular complication.

5. A: *Neisseria gonorrhoeae* is a gram-negative cocci.

6. D: *Staphylococcus aureus* is a gram-positive cocci.

7. B: The new onset of urinary incontinence may require additional medical assessment.

8. B: The suicide plan may have been decided.

9. D: *Streptobacillus moniliformis* is linked to abscesses, bacteremia, and endocarditis.

10. D: Do not administer pain medication or start a central line without MD orders.

11. A: Negative culture results would indicate absence of infection.

12. A: Purse lip breathing will help decrease the volume of air expelled by increased bronchial airways.

13. B: The Mantoux is the most accurate test to determine the presence of TB.

14. A: The frontal lobe is responsible for behavior and emotions.

15. C: >10cm/H(2)0 may indicate a condition of pericarditis

16. A: CBAN, cold, burn, ache, numbness

17. A: Theophylline toxicity may be occurring.

18. D: Respiratory alkalosis-elevated pH, and low carbon dioxide levels, no compensation noted.

19. B: Syphilis is linked to *Treponema pallidum.*
20. B: Fainting and hypotension can be caused by Tricyclics.

21. B: Palpitations and muscle weakness are found with excessive levels of Digitalis.

22. D: Inflammation of cellular tissue associated with a fever most likely indicates cellulitis.
23. A: Breath sounds would be softer.

24. B: All of the clinical signs indicate a hyperglycemic condition.

25. D: Anxiety is a clinical sign associated with respiratory acidosis.

26. D: <200 T4 cells/deciliter

27. A: The patient is at high risk of developing increased intracranial pressure (ICP).

28. B: Myocardial infarction may be associated with SOB and muscle weakness.

29. C: Muscle weakness in the lower extremities is found in acute cases of Guillain-Barre' Syndrome.

30. A: All of the others are RNA related viruses.

31. A: LOC is the most critical indicator of impaired neurological capabilities.

32. D: Streptococcus pneumoniae linked to otitis, arthritis, sinusitis, and pneumonia.

33. B: Unilateral pupil changes indicate changes in ICP.

34. D: Left sided heart failure exhibits signs of pulmonary compromise (SOB).

35. A: Edema in the lower extremities may indicate a Premarin (over-dosage).

36. A: The patient should keep the leg straight for at least 4 hours.

37. D: Digitalis can cause all of the listed symptoms.

38. A: Hypotension may be result of over correction of a hypertensive condition.

39. C: Procardia can provide the quickest relief of ischemic chest pain that is severe in this case.

40. A: Diuretics can disturb the sodium and potassium balance resulting in cardiac complications. An ECG is not indicated without evidence of cardiac conditions.

41. C: Calcium is the most recognized osteoporosis treatment.

42. D: Atropine encourages increased rate of conduction in the AV node.

43. B: Lidocaine Hydrochloride can cause fatigue and confusion if an over dosage occurs

44. D: Tachycardia, hypertension, and bronchodilation can all occur with Albuterol.

45. B: The bicarbonate value is below normal, indicating a condition of metabolic acidosis.

46. B: All of the listed signs and symptoms match up with a midbrain lesion.

47. B: The facial nerve (VII) is motor to the face and sensory to the anterior tongue.

48. B: 60-115 mg/dl is standard range for serum glucose levels.

49. A: All of the signs and symptoms match up with a lesion in the internal capsule.

50. B: Anemia and fever are associated with Zidovudine's side effects.

51. A: Both angina and hypotension are associated with Norvasc's side effects.

52. B: Elevated pH and low CO2 level indicate respiratory alkalosis, no compensation is noted.

53. A: Cognitive changes may include confusion and disorientation.

54. D: Flexeril is a muscle relaxant for acute muscle pain and spasms.

55. C: Pitressin is a hormone replacement medication.

56. D: Compulsive behavior does not indicate congenital heart defect.

57. B: All of the signs and symptoms match up with a lesion in the pons.

58. C: Venous capacity increases with morphine use.

59. D: 1.0-1.2 mEq/L is considered standard therapeutic range for patient care.

60. C: C6 Nerve Root intervates the wrist extensors and is sensory to the lateral forearm.

61. D: A-C are associated side effects of Tegretol.

62. D: A-C are associated side effects of Klonapin.

63. D: A-C are associated with diabetes mellitus.

64. A: The head of the proximal fibula is in close proximity to the peroneal nerve.

65. C: A straight line of pull is indicated with Buck's traction.

66. B: Supination- "Holding a bowl of soup in your hand."

67. B: Beta cells secrete insulin.

68. D: Insulin is not required in continuous treatment for every Type II diabetic.

69. C: Acinar cells create exocrine secretions.

70. C: Each lower extremity is scored as 18% according to the Rule of Nines.

71. A: The shock phase is considered the first 24-48 hours in wound management.

72. B: Sagittal motion occurs in the midline plane of the body.

73. B: Meningiomas tend to be encapsulated and found outside of actual brain tissue. Meningiomas are also usually benign and slow growing.

74. C: Acutely psychotic patients will disrupt group activities.

75. B: Muscle spasms and restlessness are side effects of Haldol

Secret Key #1 - Time is Your Greatest Enemy

Pace Yourself

Wear a watch. At the beginning of the test, check the time (or start a chronometer on your watch to count the minutes), and check the time after every few questions to make sure you are "on schedule."

If you are forced to speed up, do it efficiently. Usually one or more answer choices can be eliminated without too much difficulty. Above all, don't panic. Don't speed up and just begin guessing at random choices. By pacing yourself, and continually monitoring your progress against your watch, you will always know exactly how far ahead or behind you are with your available time. If you find that you are one minute behind on the test, don't skip one question without spending any time on it, just to catch back up. Take 15 fewer seconds on the next four questions, and after four questions you'll have caught back up. Once you catch back up, you can continue working each problem at your normal pace.

Furthermore, don't dwell on the problems that you were rushed on. If a problem was taking up too much time and you made a hurried guess, it must be difficult. The difficult questions are the ones you are most likely to miss anyway, so it isn't a big loss. It is better to end with more time than you need than to run out of time.

Lastly, sometimes it is beneficial to slow down if you are constantly getting ahead of time. You are always more likely to catch a careless mistake by working more slowly than quickly, and among very high-scoring test takers (those who are likely to have lots of time left over), careless errors affect the score more than mastery of material.

Secret Key #2 - Guessing is not Guesswork

You probably know that guessing is a good idea. Unlike other standardized tests, there is no penalty for getting a wrong answer. Even if you have no idea about a question, you still have a 20-25% chance of getting it right.

Most test takers do not understand the impact that proper guessing can have on their score. Unless you score extremely high, guessing will significantly contribute to your final score.

Monkeys Take the Test

What most test takers don't realize is that to insure that 20-25% chance, you have to guess randomly. If you put 20 monkeys in a room to take this test, assuming they answered once per question and behaved themselves, on average they would get 20-25% of the questions correct. Put 20 test takers in the room, and the average will be much lower among guessed questions. Why?

1. The test writers intentionally write deceptive answer choices that "look" right. A test taker has no idea about a question, so he picks the "best looking" answer, which is often wrong. The monkey has no idea what looks good and what doesn't, so it will consistently be right about 20-25% of the time.

2. Test takers will eliminate answer choices from the guessing pool based on a hunch or intuition. Simple but correct answers often get excluded, leaving a 0% chance of being correct. The monkey has no clue, and often gets lucky with the best choice.

This is why the process of elimination endorsed by most test courses is flawed and detrimental to your performance. Test takers don't guess; they make an ignorant stab in the dark that is usually worse than random.

$5 Challenge

Let me introduce one of the most valuable ideas of this course—the $5 challenge:

You only mark your "best guess" if you are willing to bet $5 on it.
You only eliminate choices from guessing if you are willing to bet $5 on it.

Why $5? Five dollars is an amount of money that is small yet not insignificant, and can really add up fast (20 questions could cost you $100). Likewise, each answer choice on one question of the test will have a small impact on your overall score, but it can really add up to a lot of points in the end.

The process of elimination IS valuable. The following shows your chance of guessing it right:

If you eliminate wrong answer choices until only this many remain:	Chance of getting it correct:
1	100%
2	50%
3	33%

However, if you accidentally eliminate the right answer or go on a hunch for an incorrect answer, your chances drop dramatically—to 0%. By guessing among all the answer choices, you are GUARANTEED to have a shot at the right answer.

That's why the $5 test is so valuable. If you give up the advantage and safety of a pure guess, it had better be worth the risk.

What we still haven't covered is how to be sure that whatever guess you make is truly random. Here's the easiest way:

Always pick the first answer choice among those remaining.

Such a technique means that you have decided, **before you see a single test question**, exactly how you are going to guess, and since the order of choices tells you nothing about which one is correct, this guessing technique is perfectly random.

This section is not meant to scare you away from making educated guesses or eliminating choices; you just need to define when a choice is worth eliminating. The $5 test, along with a pre-defined random guessing strategy, is the best way to make sure you reap all of the benefits of guessing.

Secret Key #3 - Practice Smarter, Not Harder

Many test takers delay the test preparation process because they dread the awful amounts of practice time they think necessary to succeed on the test. We have refined an effective method that will take you only a fraction of the time.

There are a number of "obstacles" in the path to success. Among these are answering questions, finishing in time, and mastering test-taking strategies. All must be executed on the day of the test at peak performance, or your score will suffer. The test is a mental marathon that has a large impact on your future.

Just like a marathon runner, it is important to work your way up to the full challenge. So first you just worry about questions, and then time, and finally strategy:

Success Strategy

1. Find a good source for practice tests.
2. If you are willing to make a larger time investment, consider using more than one study guide. Often the different approaches of multiple authors will help you "get" difficult concepts.
3. Take a practice test with no time constraints, with all study helps, "open book." Take your time with questions and focus on applying strategies.
4. Take a practice test with time constraints, with all guides, "open book."
5. Take a final practice test without open material and with time limits.

If you have time to take more practice tests, just repeat step 5. By gradually exposing yourself to the full rigors of the test environment, you will condition your mind to the stress of test day and maximize your success.

Secret Key #4 - Prepare, Don't Procrastinate

Let me state an obvious fact: if you take the test three times, you will probably get three different scores. This is due to the way you feel on test day, the level of preparedness you have, and the version of the test you see. Despite the test writers' claims to the contrary, some versions of the test WILL be easier for you than others.

Since your future depends so much on your score, you should maximize your chances of success. In order to maximize the likelihood of success, you've got to prepare in advance. This means taking practice tests and spending time learning the information and test taking strategies you will need to succeed.

Never go take the actual test as a "practice" test, expecting that you can just take it again if you need to. Take all the practice tests you can on your own, but when you go to take the official test, be prepared, be focused, and do your best the first time!

Secret Key #5 - Test Yourself

Everyone knows that time is money. There is no need to spend too much of your time or too little of your time preparing for the test. You should only spend as much of your precious time preparing as is necessary for you to get the score you need.

Once you have taken a practice test under real conditions of time constraints, then you will know if you are ready for the test or not.
If you have scored extremely high the first time that you take the practice test, then there is not much point in spending countless hours studying. You are already there.

Benchmark your abilities by retaking practice tests and seeing how much you have improved. Once you consistently score high enough to guarantee success, then you are ready.

If you have scored well below where you need, then knuckle down and begin studying in earnest. Check your improvement regularly through the use of practice tests under real conditions. Above all, don't worry, panic, or give up. The key is perseverance!

Then, when you go to take the test, remain confident and remember how well you did on the practice tests. If you can score high enough on a practice test, then you can do the same on the real thing.

General Strategies

The most important thing you can do is to ignore your fears and jump into the test immediately. Do not be overwhelmed by any strange-sounding terms. You have to jump into the test like jumping into a pool—all at once is the easiest way.

Make Predictions
As you read and understand the question, try to guess what the answer will be. Remember that several of the answer choices are wrong, and once you begin reading them, your mind will immediately become cluttered with answer choices designed to throw you off. Your mind is typically the most focused immediately after you have read the question and digested its contents. If you can, try to predict what the correct answer will be. You may be surprised at what you can predict.

Quickly scan the choices and see if your prediction is in the listed answer choices. If it is, then you can be quite confident that you have the right answer. It still won't hurt to check the other answer choices, but most of the time, you've got it!

Answer the Question
It may seem obvious to only pick answer choices that answer the question, but the test writers can create some excellent answer choices that are wrong. Don't pick an answer just because it sounds right, or you believe it to be true. It MUST answer the question. Once you've made your selection, always go back and check it against the question and make sure that you didn't misread the question and that the answer choice does answer the question posed.

Benchmark
After you read the first answer choice, decide if you think it sounds correct or not. If it doesn't, move on to the next answer choice. If it does, mentally mark that answer choice. This doesn't mean that you've definitely selected it as your answer choice, it just means that it's the best you've seen thus far. Go ahead and read the next choice. If the next choice is worse than the one you've already selected, keep going to

the next answer choice. If the next choice is better than the choice you've already selected, mentally mark the new answer choice as your best guess.

The first answer choice that you select becomes your standard. Every other answer choice must be benchmarked against that standard. That choice is correct until proven otherwise by another answer choice beating it out. Once you've decided that no other answer choice seems as good, do one final check to ensure that your answer choice answers the question posed.

Valid Information
Don't discount any of the information provided in the question. Every piece of information may be necessary to determine the correct answer. None of the information in the question is there to throw you off (while the answer choices will certainly have information to throw you off). If two seemingly unrelated topics are discussed, don't ignore either. You can be confident there is a relationship, or it wouldn't be included in the question, and you are probably going to have to determine what is that relationship to find the answer.

Avoid "Fact Traps"
Don't get distracted by a choice that is factually true. Your search is for the answer that answers the question. Stay focused and don't fall for an answer that is true but irrelevant. Always go back to the question and make sure you're choosing an answer that actually answers the question and is not just a true statement. An answer can be factually correct, but it MUST answer the question asked. Additionally, two answers can both be seemingly correct, so be sure to read all of the answer choices, and make sure that you get the one that BEST answers the question.

Milk the Question
Some of the questions may throw you completely off. They might deal with a subject you have not been exposed to, or one that you haven't reviewed in years. While your lack of knowledge about the subject will be a hindrance, the question itself can give you many clues that will help you find the correct answer. Read the question carefully and look for clues. Watch particularly for adjectives and nouns describing difficult terms or words that you don't recognize. Regardless of whether you completely understand a word or not, replacing it with a synonym, either provided or one you more familiar with, may help you to understand what the questions are asking. Rather than wracking your mind about specific detailed information concerning a difficult term or word, try to use mental substitutes that are easier to understand.

The Trap of Familiarity
Don't just choose a word because you recognize it. On difficult questions, you may not recognize a number of words in the answer choices. The test writers don't put "make-believe" words on the test, so don't think that just because you only recognize all the words in one answer choice that that answer choice must be correct. If you only recognize words in one answer choice, then focus on that one. Is it correct? Try your best to determine if it is correct. If it is, that's great. If not, eliminate it. Each word and answer choice you eliminate increases your chances of getting the question correct, even if you then have to guess among the unfamiliar choices.

Eliminate Answers
Eliminate choices as soon as you realize they are wrong. But be careful! Make sure you consider all of the possible answer choices. Just because one appears right, doesn't mean that the next one won't be even better! The test writers will usually put more than one good answer choice for every question, so read all of them. Don't worry if you are stuck between two that seem right. By getting down to just two remaining possible choices, your odds are now 50/50. Rather than wasting too much time, play the odds.

You are guessing, but guessing wisely because you've been able to knock out some of the answer choices that you know are wrong. If you are eliminating choices and realize that the last answer choice you are left with is also obviously wrong, don't panic. Start over and consider each choice again. There may easily be something that you missed the first time and will realize on the second pass.

Tough Questions
If you are stumped on a problem or it appears too hard or too difficult, don't waste time. Move on! Remember though, if you can quickly check for obviously incorrect answer choices, your chances of guessing correctly are greatly improved. Before you completely give up, at least try to knock out a couple of possible answers. Eliminate what you can and then guess at the remaining answer choices before moving on.

Brainstorm
If you get stuck on a difficult question, spend a few seconds quickly brainstorming. Run through the complete list of possible answer choices. Look at each choice and ask yourself, "Could this answer the question satisfactorily?" Go through each answer choice and consider it independently of the others. By systematically going through all possibilities, you may find something that you would otherwise overlook. Remember though that when you get stuck, it's important to try to keep moving.

Read Carefully
Understand the problem. Read the question and answer choices carefully. Don't miss the question because you misread the terms. You have plenty of time to read each question thoroughly and make sure you understand what is being asked. Yet a happy medium must be attained, so don't waste too much time. You must read carefully, but efficiently.

Face Value
When in doubt, use common sense. Always accept the situation in the problem at face value. Don't read too much into it. These problems will not require you to make huge leaps of logic. The test writers aren't trying to throw you off with a cheap trick. If you have to go beyond creativity and make a leap of logic in order to have an answer choice answer the question, then you should look at the other answer choices. Don't overcomplicate the problem by creating theoretical relationships or explanations that will warp time or space. These are normal problems rooted in reality. It's just that the applicable relationship or explanation may not be readily apparent and you have to figure things out. Use your common sense to interpret anything that isn't clear.

Prefixes
If you're having trouble with a word in the question or answer choices, try dissecting it. Take advantage of every clue that the word might include. Prefixes and suffixes can be a huge help. Usually they allow you to determine a basic meaning. Pre- means before, post- means after, pro - is positive, de- is negative. From these prefixes and suffixes, you can get an idea of the general meaning of the word and try to put it into context. Beware though of any traps. Just because con- is the opposite of pro-, doesn't necessarily mean congress is the opposite of progress!

Hedge Phrases
Watch out for critical hedge phrases, led off with words such as "likely," "may," "can," "sometimes," "often," "almost," "mostly," "usually," "generally," "rarely," and "sometimes." Question writers insert these hedge phrases to cover every possibility. Often an answer choice will be wrong simply because it leaves no room for exception. Unless the situation calls for them, avoid answer choices that have definitive words like "exactly," and "always."

Switchback Words

Stay alert for "switchbacks." These are the words and phrases frequently used to alert you to shifts in thought. The most common switchback word is "but." Others include "although," "however," "nevertheless," "on the other hand," "even though," "while," "in spite of," "despite," and "regardless of."

New Information

Correct answer choices will rarely have completely new information included. Answer choices typically are straightforward reflections of the material asked about and will directly relate to the question. If a new piece of information is included in an answer choice that doesn't even seem to relate to the topic being asked about, then that answer choice is likely incorrect. All of the information needed to answer the question is usually provided for you in the question. You should not have to make guesses that are unsupported or choose answer choices that require unknown information that cannot be reasoned from what is given.

Time Management

On technical questions, don't get lost on the technical terms. Don't spend too much time on any one question. If you don't know what a term means, then odds are you aren't going to get much further since you don't have a dictionary. You should be able to immediately recognize whether or not you know a term. If you don't, work with the other clues that you have—the other answer choices and terms provided—but don't waste too much time trying to figure out a difficult term that you don't know.

Contextual Clues

Look for contextual clues. An answer can be right but not the correct answer. The contextual clues will help you find the answer that is most right and is correct. Understand the context in which a phrase or statement is made. This will help you make important distinctions.

Don't Panic

Panicking will not answer any questions for you; therefore, it isn't helpful. When you first see the question, if your mind goes blank, take a deep breath. Force yourself to mechanically go through the steps of solving the problem using the strategies you've learned.

Pace Yourself

Don't get clock fever. It's easy to be overwhelmed when you're looking at a page full of questions, your mind is full of random thoughts and feeling confused, and the clock is ticking down faster than you would like. Calm down and maintain the pace that you have set for yourself. As long as you are on track by monitoring your pace, you are guaranteed to have enough time for yourself. When you get to the last few minutes of the test, it may seem like you won't have enough time left, but if you only have as many questions as you should have left at that point, then you're right on track!

Answer Selection

The best way to pick an answer choice is to eliminate all of those that are wrong, until only one is left and confirm that is the correct answer. Sometimes though, an answer choice may immediately look right. Be careful! Take a second to make sure that the other choices are not equally obvious. Don't make a hasty mistake. There are only two times that you should stop before checking other answers. First is when you are positive that the answer choice you have selected is correct. Second is when time is almost out and you have to make a quick guess!

Check Your Work

Since you will probably not know every term listed and the answer to every question, it is important that you get credit for the ones that you do know. Don't miss any questions through careless mistakes. If at all possible, try to take a second to look back over your answer selection and make sure you've selected the correct answer choice and haven't made a costly careless mistake (such as marking an answer choice that you didn't mean to mark). The time it takes for this quick double check should more than pay for itself in caught mistakes.

Beware of Directly Quoted Answers
Sometimes an answer choice will repeat word for word a portion of the question or reference section. However, beware of such exact duplication. It may be a trap! More than likely, the correct choice will paraphrase or summarize a point, rather than being exactly the same wording.

Slang
Scientific sounding answers are better than slang ones. An answer choice that begins "To compare the outcomes..." is much more likely to be correct than one that begins "Because some people insisted..."

Extreme Statements
Avoid wild answers that throw out highly controversial ideas that are proclaimed as established fact. An answer choice that states the "process should be used in certain situations, if..." is much more likely to be correct than one that states the "process should be discontinued completely." The first is a calm rational statement and doesn't even make a definitive, uncompromising stance, using a hedge word "if" to provide wiggle room, whereas the second choice is a radical idea and far more extreme.

Answer Choice Families
When you have two or more answer choices that are direct opposites or parallels, one of them is usually the correct answer. For instance, if one answer choice states "x increases" and another answer choice states "x decreases" or "y increases," then those two or three answer choices are very similar in construction and fall into the same family of answer choices. A family of answer choices consists of two or three answer choices, very similar in construction, but often with directly opposite meanings. Usually the correct answer choice will be in that family of answer choices. The "odd man out" or answer choice that doesn't seem to fit the parallel construction of the other answer choices is more likely to be incorrect.

Special Report: Additional Bonus Material

Due to our efforts to try to keep this book to a manageable length, we've created a link that will give you access to all of your additional bonus material.

Please visit http://www.mometrix.com/bonus948/pance to access the information.